People with Epilepsy

HOW THEY CAN BE HELPED

Mary V. Laidlaw SRN
Rehabilitation Adviser, The Epilepsy Centre,
Quarrier's Homes, Bridge of Weir, Scotland

John Laidlaw FRCP (Edin)
Consultant Physician, The Epilepsy Centre,
Quarrier's Homes, Bridge of Weir, Scotland

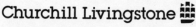
Churchill Livingstone

EDINBURGH LONDON MELBOURNE AND NEW YORK 1984

CHURCHILL LIVINGSTONE
Medical Division of Longman Group Limited

Distributed in the United States of America by Churchill Livingstone Inc., 1560 Broadway, New York, N.Y. 10036, and by associated companies, branches and representatives throughout the world.

First published 1984

ISBN 0 443 02810 9

British Library Cataloguing in Publication Data
Laidlaw, Mary V.
  People with epilepsy.
  1. Epilepsy
  I. Title   II. Laidlaw, John
  616.8′53   RC372

Library of Congress Cataloging in Publication Data
Laidlaw, Mary V.
  People with epilepsy.
  Includes index.
  1. Epilepsy. I. Laidlaw, John Patrick. II. Title.
[DNLM: 1. Epilepsy. WL 385 L185p]
RC372.L285   1983   616.8′53   83-15175

Printed in Singapore by
Huntsmen Offset Printing Ltd.

People with
Epilepsy

To
Dr Denis Williams
from whom we have both learned so much

Preface

This book completes a triad of books about epilepsy with which we have been associated: all published by Churchill Livingstone: *Epilepsy Explained* (Laidlaw and Laidlaw, 2nd printing, 1982) a short simple book written primarily for those with epilepsy and their families: and *The Textbook of Epilepsy* (Eds. Laidlaw and Richens, 2nd edition, 1982) a definitive text for specialists in all those disciplines concerned with epilepsy. *People with Epilepsy* is written for all those whose work involves helping such people: general practitioners, nurses, social workers, teachers, clergymen and many others. It should be of value also to people with epilepsy themselves and their families.

We have tried to avoid medical jargon but we have used ordinary medical terms when they are appropriate. Since some readers may not be familiar with these terms we have included a glossary to explain them. The first time that a word in the glossary appears in the text it is printed in italics. In Appendix A we have listed the main antiepileptic drugs with the official (generic) and some of the proprietary names with a note of the names of the more important drugs in other countries. In Appendix B we give the names and addresses of the Epilepsy Associations in the U.K. These Associations provide valuable up-to-date information on such subjects as: Epilepsy

Associations in other countries, immigration restrictions on people with epilepsy, and antiepileptic drug names in foreign countries not mentioned in Appendix A.

Throughout the book we have included 14 illustrative stories, or Personal Situations. These stories are all based on real cases. We hope that they will be memorable and that they will help to emphasize some of the points of importance which we have tried to make.

Finally we would like to acknowledge the tremendous help which we have had from our secretary Mrs Dunbar, from Miss MacGilchrist who has helped with the typing, from Miss Maureen Simpson, a resident at our Epilepsy Centre, for her rough drafts of some of the illustrations, and from Mrs Amos, Chief EEG Technician who selected suitable specimens for the EEG figures.

Bridge of Weir,   M.V.L.
Scotland, 1984   J.L.

Contents

Introduction

EPILEPSY IS AN ENIGMA

The practice of medicine attempts ideally and somewhat optimistically to cure disease, but more often and more realistically succeeds in alleviating symptoms, and always should be able to provide comfort and support to those in distress. Throughout history it is fair to say that, by and large, doctors have been professional people and honest people: whether befeathered witch doctors, elegant top-hatted Victorian physicians, or over-casually dressed professors (call me 'Tom') surrounded by the computerized hardware of the late twentieth century. Those who are professional and honest may be deemed so because their practice of medicine—their treatment of disease—is not frivolous or haphazard, but rather based on their understanding of the cause of disease. Thus the history of medicine is not so much the history of treatments as the history of concepts of causes: the honest professional offers treatment appropriate to the cause of the illness. As one moves from the primitive to the sophisticated, one moves from evil spirits, to Gods and Devils, through phlegms and fluxes, to germs and the too often invisible viruses, to the immune responses reacting to the invasion of foreign proteins, to the hugely complex influence of chemical mediators of our

physical functions, and perhaps back again to the little understood influence of the mind.

It has been suggested with much truth that the history of
epilepsy provides a microcosm of the history of medicine.
Certainly, epilepsy, once termed the Sacred Disease, might
more accurately be described as the most Ancient Disease.
Even before the well-known references in the Bible, Hippo-
crates in 400BC attributed seizures to a disorder of the brain,
and some 6000 years ago reference is made in the Babylonian
Code of Hammurabi to febrile convulsions and the laws perti-
nent to the marriage and employment of 'epileptics'. Over
these many centuries there have been diverse postulates as to
the cause of this enigmatic disorder, ranging from the reasonable to the bizarrely irrational, and consequently suggestions
as to treatment ranging from the harmless to the horrific
(Temkin, 1971). Now, at the end of the twentieth century, there
has been a huge increase in our understanding of causes, and
so an improvement in our methods of treatment: but the enigma remains.

What then is the enigma?

We need to consider three questions: what happens during
a seizure? why do some people have recurrent seizures (have
epilepsy)? why do those with epilepsy have seizures when
they do (what is the proximate precipitant)?

What happens during a seizure?

The functions of our bodies are controlled in large measure by
the nervous system: the brain, the spinal cord, and the nerves
which run from the spinal cord to the muscles and from the
sense organs inwards to the spinal cord and the brain. This
control is effected by exceedingly minute electrical impulses
which in turn release a variety of complex chemical substances. The latter cannot be measured during life and will
not be considered in this book. The electrical impulses in the
brain, when magnified some million or so times, can be recorded on the *electroencephalograph* (*EEG*) and may be visu-
alized either on paper or on an oscillograph (like a TV screen).
EEG records have added a lot to our understanding of what
happens during an epileptic seizure. In particular, it is usually
possible to determine whether or not a fit—an observed event

of altered behaviour—is or is not accompanied by an electrical event which will help to decide whether or not the fit is an epileptic seizure. We will consider without technical detail the usefulness and limitations of the EEG record. Most people with suspected epilepsy will have EEG tests, which often they find mysterious if not frightening, and it is important that those, including their GPs, whose job it is to help them, should have an understanding of the test.

Why do some people have recurrent seizures?

We are nearer to an answer to this question. Damage to the brain may result in an area of irritation from which a seizure may develop. However, not all people with similar brain damage develop epilepsy and some people have seizures without any demonstrable brain damage. We have to postulate, therefore, the additional factor of a degree of brain sensitivity with which a person is born, and which may or may not be hereditary.

What is the proximate precipitant?

Here lies the great enigma, and because an enigma is always a challenge this is the fascination that epilepsy has had for doctors and paramedical workers throughout the ages.

There are a few clear precipitants: the sudden withdrawal or reduction in antiepileptic drugs (or alcohol), or, especially in children, abnormalities of blood constituents. A number of possible or probable precipitants have been suggested, such as excessive physical or mental stress.

However, the enigma remains. Why should someone living a sedate and ordered life, whose treatment has remained constant, have three seizures in a year: at 3.15 p.m. on January 17th, 11.00 a.m. on March 20th and at 8.00 p.m. on September 1st, rather than at 3.20 p.m. on January 18th, 10.00 a.m. on March 19th or at midnight on Christmas Eve? The great majority of seizures occur for no apparent reason: they are enigmas. We might be excused if we gave up and, with humility, had recourse to the ancient concept that they were provoked by the supernatural. If we are not prepared to accept such defeat, we must suggest that the proximate precipitant is more mundane: that it is the result of some change in environment. The person with epilepsy is exposed to two environments. There is the Internal Environment of the various chemical substances in the blood and body fluids, which includes the drugs given for control of epilepsy; and the External Environment, which includes all the social and psychological influences of the world in which a person lives. The internal environment is the province of the scientist and the informed doctor. The external environment is, however, the province of all those who are concerned with helping the person with epilepsy. It is for all such people that this book is written. Since epilepsy is not just a problem for doctors, it seems so important that other professional disciplines should have a sufficient understanding of medical matters, so that they are in the position to co-operate with medical advice, rather than that they should be expected to accept uncritically what doctors tell them to do.

REFERENCE

Temkin O 1971 The falling sickness. The Johns Hopkins Press, Baltimore & London

1

The population of people with epilepsy

One in every 200 of the population has epilepsy, i.e. has recurrent fits. Why the one and not the other 199?

Whatever the preceding or consequential biochemical events (which we have suggested are beyond the scope of this book), the seizure is accompanied by an electrical event which can be measured and seen (Fig. 1.1). This electrical event arises in and can be recorded from the brain. As the great British neurologist Hughlings Jackson anticipated about a hundred years ago, it is the result of 'an excessive and a disorderly discharge of nervous tissue'.

This catastrophic event in the brain may arise primarily in the brain, in which case it is considered to be epilepsy, or it may arise because of disorders outside the brain which affect brain function, in which case it is not usually considered as epilepsy.

Fits caused by events outside the brain.

There are a large number of disorders which so affect the internal environment of the body (the blood and tissue fluids) that in turn the internal environment of the brain is so disturbed as to result in a fit. The precipitant of the fit is known and, if it can be avoided or eliminated, the patient will not be subject to recurrent fits and so may not be considered as

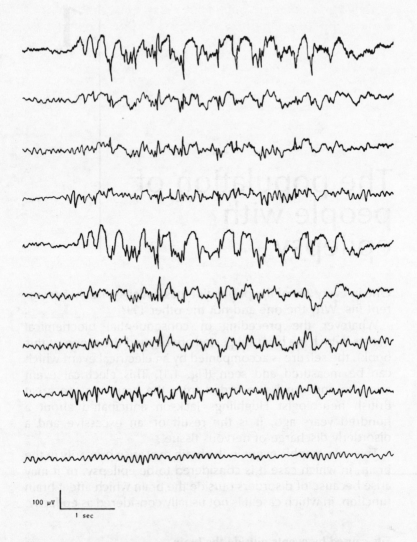

100 µV

1 sec

Fig. 1.1 A paroxysm of about 5 seconds with a normal record before and after.

In all the EEG figures the vertical line in the left hand bottom corner represents the deflection produced by 100 microvolts, and the horizontal line the distance that the paper moves in one second. In all figures except 3.5. the extra line at the bottom is an example of a normal record. In this figure and 2.8, 3.5, 3.8. to 3.11, and 12.1, the first four lines come from the right side from the front to the back, and the lower four lines from the left side.

suffering from epilepsy. Since these precipitants are of interest some of the more important will be considered.

1. Oxygen lack

Oxygen is essential for the normal working of all body tissues. It is carried in the blood which in turn is pumped round the body by the heart. The brain has very high oxygen needs and, if there is a degree of heart failure, the brain will suffer and the patient will become confused. If there is a sudden complete failure of the heart's action, loss of brain oxygen may result in a fit.

In elderly people the heart may stop altogether, or it may beat so rapidly that it is unable to pump blood effectively. These conditions are treatable and so fits need not be recurrent. Younger people are liable to faints in which there is an expansion of the blood vessels in the lower parts of the body so that there is not enough blood left for the brain. The immediate effect is loss of consciousness, the person falls, and, being horizontal, blood returns to the brain and there is quick recovery. If for some reason he does not or cannot fall, the brain is deprived of blood for so long that he has a fit. This may happen to a soldier on parade, who inadvisedly is supported in the upright position by his neighbours.

2. Glucose lack

Glucose is essential for normal brain function. It is not uncommon for small infants to have very low levels of blood glucose (*hypoglycaemia*) and, as a result, for them to have fits. They do not suffer from epilepsy because if the hypoglycaemia is corrected the fits stop. Insulin is well known as the drug which controls excessive levels of glucose in the blood (hyperglycaemia). Overdosage with insulin may result in severe hypoglycaemia and resulting fits. Certain severe forms of mental illness have for many years been treated with *electroconvulsive therapy* (*ECT*) (passing electric currents through the brain to cause seizures). At one time there was the alternative of insulin therapy when similar artificial fits were produced by increasing doses of insulin: these patients had fits but they did not suffer from epilepsy.

3. Kidney failure

The kidneys get rid of waste products from the blood. When they fail there is an accumulation of these waste products and some of them affect the brain and cause fits.

4. Drug withdrawal

The sudden withdrawal of drugs, for example phenobarbitone, may result in fits. Nowadays phenobarbitone is seldom given except to those with epilepsy. However, if a pregnant woman with epilepsy is being treated with phenobarbitone some of this will get into the blood of the unborn baby. After birth the infant's supply of phenobarbitone is cut off suddenly and he may have fits. He has been born with his mother's phenobarbitone: he has not inherited his mother's epilepsy.

The role that alcohol plays in epilepsy is uncertain. However, if someone habitually drinking heavily, stops suddenly, fits may occur as one of the effects of withdrawal.

5. Convulsant drugs

Certain drugs, particularly some tranquillizers and antidepressants, are known to exacerbate fits in people with epilepsy. It is probable that some cause fits in those who would otherwise not be subject to recurrent fits—who would not otherwise have epilepsy.

Figure 1.2 represents a normal brain surrounded by a circle which may be considered as enclosing a representation of the internal environment which is clear of any of those severe disorders which may cause fits. The patient has no fits and, of course, has no epilepsy.

Figure 1.3 represents a normal brain but one which is surrounded by an internal environment sufficiently disordered to precipitate fits. The patient has fits but does not suffer from epilepsy, since if the internal environment can be returned to normal there will be no recurrent fits.

This explanation of the effects of severe disorders of the internal environment is probably an over-simplification and it is worthwhile considering it further. It was suggested in the Introduction that there were two factors which combined to cause recurrent fits—brain sensitivity and brain damage. Might these factors also determine whether or not internal environmental factors did or did not cause fits—even if not epilepsy? The drug leptazol is used to differentiate the type of fit from which a person with epilepsy suffers. A relatively small dose of leptazol will cause a fit in someone suffering from epilepsy, but a sufficient dose will cause a fit in someone who does not suffer from epilepsy. Perhaps there is a threshold for the production of fits which depends on the degree of brain sensitivity and/or brain damage. Not all those with kidney failure have fits, nor all those deprived of oxygen or glucose. Perhaps, we should consider that those who do, have a lower epileptic threshold, and although they cannot be considered as suffering from epilepsy, may be more liable to develop fits than the rest of the population. Not only does this concept have practical importance but also it may help to dispel the pejorative distinction between 'epileptics' and the rest of us.

We can, therefore, extend the brain–internal environment diagrams. Figure 1.4 represents someone with a very high threshold who, subject to extreme stress, has a fit.

Figure 1.5 represents someone with a lower threshold due to some brain sensitivity (shown by dots) who, subject to moderate stress, has a fit. May this person be more liable to epilepsy?

Similarly Figure 1.6 represents another with a lower threshold due to some brain damage (shown by hatched area) who also may be more liable to epilepsy.

Finally, some of the internal environmental factors which precipitate fits in those who do not suffer from epilepsy, may be important in precipitating fits in those who do. Deep breathing, which may occur in people who are fussed, can alter the blood gases in the direction of reducing the oxygen to the brain, and thus might possibly precipitate a seizure.

Fits due to primary brain disorder

Since in adults such fits are usually recurrent, they may be considered as constituting epilepsy. *Febrile convulsions* which occur in young children at the time of a high temperature do not constitute epilepsy, and are due to a combination of a primary brain disorder and the impact of a stress outwith the brain.

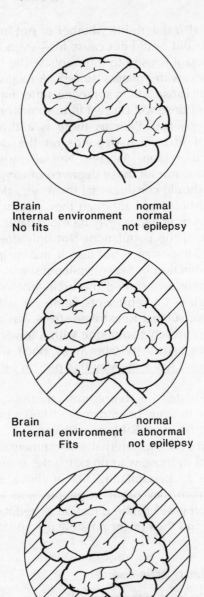

Fig. 1.2

Brain	normal
Internal environment	normal
No fits	not epilepsy

Fig. 1.3

Brain	normal
Internal environment	abnormal
Fits	not epilepsy

Fig. 1.4

Brain	normal
Internal environment	very abnormal
Fits	not epilepsy

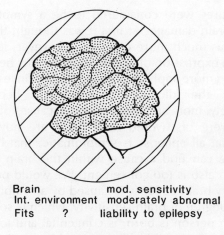

Fig. 1.5

Brain		mod. sensitivity
Int. environment		moderately abnormal
Fits	?	liability to epilepsy

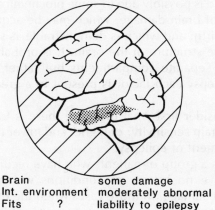

Fig. 1.6

Brain		some damage
Int. environment		moderately abnormal
Fits	?	liability to epilepsy

Figs. 1.2 to 1.6 Diagrams to show the effects of the internal environment, brain sensitivity and brain damage on the occurrence of fits. The area between the brain diagram and the circle represents the internal environment. Hatching shows the degree of abnormality of the internal environment. Dots in the brain diagram represent brain sensitivity, cross-hatching brain damage.

Not so long ago epilepsy was subdivided into two convenient compartments: *idiopathic epilepsy*, which really meant that no cause could be found in the sense of obvious brain damage, and which was considered, therefore, to be due to an inherited liability to seizures: and *symptomatic epilepsy*, when seizures were considered to be a symptom of some apparent brain damage. At first it was thought that idiopathic epilepsy was much more common. However, idiopathic was in effect an expression of 'we don't know why he has fits', and as more and more sophisticated methods of investigation were developed, the idiopathic compartment became eroded progressively, more and more potential causes of symptomatic epilepsy were discovered, and there are now those who propose that all epilepsy is symptomatic: that if we try hard enough we can find a cause within the brain. Perhaps this explanation also is too convenient. We would propose rather that primary brain epilepsy is caused by a combination of two factors: a degree of brain sensitivity, which is something with which each person is born, is congenital and to some extent inherited, and is possibly due to some biochemical defect: and an element of brain damage, which may be acquired before, at, or after birth, and which is demonstrable as some obvious change in the structure of the brain. It is probable that there are not two separate compartments but rather that in most cases of epilepsy each factor is present to a greater or lesser extent.

Let us consider first what evidence there is for the idea of degrees of brain sensitivity: of higher and lower thresholds for the development of epilepsy.

1. There is a group of patients who have recurrent seizures but who have no history of conditions which might have caused brain damage. In those cases when the brain has been examined after death, it has not been possible to find any abnormality. Furthermore, patients in this group often have a family history of epilepsy.

2. As we have mentioned, if the convulsant drug leptazol is given to those known to have epilepsy, fits can be provoked with quite low doses. If those not suffering from epilepsy are given leptazol, fits can always be provoked if a large enough dose is given. However, there is a wide range of doses sufficient to cause seizures in such people. This suggests that even those who do not have epilepsy have a range of liability to seizures, i.e. they have different convulsive thresholds.

3. Certain forms of brain damage (or *lesions*) are very liable to cause fits: for example brain *tumours* or brain *abscesses*. However, although a brain abscess is one of the lesions most

likely to cause fits, about a quarter of patients with abscesses, wherever they may be sited in the brain, do not have seizures.

These points might suggest that it is possible for someone with a very high brain sensitivity—a very low threshold for seizures—to have epilepsy, without any evidence, which we can demonstrate presently (Fig. 1.7).

Whereas on the other hand, for the same reasons even a brain lesion most likely to cause seizures will do so only if there is some degree of brain sensitivity. Figure 1.8 would represent a patient with a brain abscess who had fits because of a measure of brain sensitivity. The patient in Figure 1.9, also

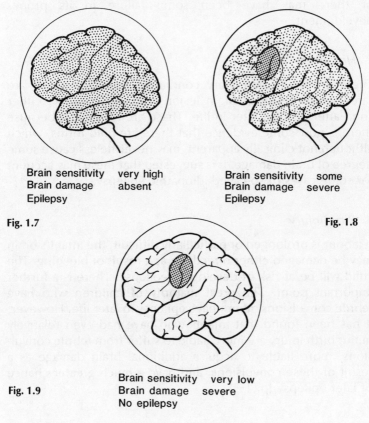

Brain sensitivity   very high
Brain damage   absent
Epilepsy

Fig. 1.7

Brain sensitivity   some
Brain damage   severe
Epilepsy

Fig. 1.8

Brain sensitivity   very low
Brain damage   severe
No epilepsy

Fig. 1.9

Figs. 1.7 to 1.9 Diagrams to show the effects of brain sensitivity and brain damage in the causation of epilepsy. As in Figs 1.2 to 1.6, dots represent brain sensitivity and cross-hatching brain damage.

with a brain abscess, would not have fits because of a high threshold for seizures—an absence of adequate brain sensitivity.

There are many lesions which damage the brain and cause epilepsy in those with a measure of brain sensitivity. We will consider those which are common or which are of special interest.

1. Congenital

The unborn baby's brain may suffer damage in the womb because of an infection from which the mother has suffered, or there may have been some failure in its proper development.

2. Hereditary

There are many hereditary conditions—most of which are rare—which result in brain lesions causing epilepsy, either soon after birth or later in life. These are of interest because there is now some evidence that there are mild forms, which although not clinically apparent, may nevertheless cause some degree of brain damage. It is suggested that these may account for some cases of so-called idiopathic epilepsy.

3. Birth injury

If labour is prolonged or particularly difficult, the infant's brain may be damaged either directly or as a result of bleeding. The child will be at risk of developing epilepsy. There is a further important point. The great majority of children who have febrile convulsions do not have epilepsy in later life. However, it has been found that infants who have had even relatively minor birth injury are more liable to suffer from febrile convulsions, more liable to acquire additional brain damage as a result of these convulsions, and have a much greater chance of later epilepsy (p. 153).

4. Infections

These may be of the brain substance (*encephalitis*) or of the membranes (*meninges*) which cover the brain (*meningitis*).

Although there have been severe epidemics of encephalitis, on the whole it is now a good deal less common than meningitis. However, it may be diagnosed less readily, and it is more difficult to treat effectively. Meningitis presents with more obvious symptoms and signs: severe headache, dislike of the light (*photophobia*), temperature and neck stiffness. Most cases can be treated successfully with antibiotics and prompt treatment reduces the risk of brain damage and later epilepsy. Meningitis in infants is much more difficult to recognize. It often presents with a seizure which may be confused with a simple febrile convulsion. If there is any doubt, infants with febrile convulsions should be admitted to hospital. The diagnosis can be established by examining the fluid surrounding the brain (*cerebrospinal fluid or c.s.f.*) (see p. 59). Brain infections may become localized to form brain abscesses. Ear infections, if not adequately treated, are an important cause of abscesses in the underlying part of the brain (the *temporal* lobe). Once a brain abscess has developed, although it can be treated either with antibiotics or by surgery, there is a high risk of later epilepsy (p. 12).

5. Direct injury

Head injuries vary enormously in severity from the trivial to the disastrous and fatal. Rather obviously, the degree of brain damage and the risk of subsequent epilepsy will be related to the severity of the injury. It is important to have some understanding of this risk in order to be able to reassure patients and their families. If a small child trips when playing, bumps his head and appears momentarily dazed, it is highly improbable that the brain will have been damaged to the extent of causing later epilepsy. However, should he do so, his mother may remember the incident, and, quite wrongly, be overwhelmed with the guilt that it was her negligence which caused his epilepsy.

Many cases of epilepsy were caused by missile injuries to the head during war. Nowadays, the commonest cause of severe head injuries is the civilian massacres which occur in our road traffic accidents.

Careful studies of epilepsy following head injury have identified factors which increase the probability of the development of established epilepsy: loss of memory for several hours after the injury (*post-traumatic amnesia*), injuries involving a fracture of the skull, injuries in which the meninges covering the brain have been penetrated, and injuries in which there has been bleeding into the brain and a clot of blood (*haematoma*) has had to be removed.

6. Brain tumours

Although children may develop brain tumours, they are unlikely to be in a part of the brain which will result in epilepsy. However, adult brain tumours cause fits in quite a high proportion of patients. Since such tumours are potentially lethal and in many cases able to be removed successfully by operation, neurologists quite rightly spend a great deal of time making sure that someone who has a fit after, say, the age of 18, does not have a causative tumour. Although their investigations are wholly proper, it is important to be able to reassure patients on two counts. Firstly, that brain tumours, although very likely to cause seizures, are not as probable a cause as the prudence of the neurologists might suggest. And secondly, that modern methods of investigation are painless, without risk of complications, and sufficiently accurate to make it possible to exclude a tumour.

7. Blood vessel (vascular) disorders

Brain damage may be caused either by the destruction of tissue by *haemorrhage* or by the death of tissue which does not get the blood it needs to survive. *Vascular* disorders are an important cause of seizure at all ages.

a. A child may be born with abnormal blood vessels over a part of the brain which in consequence shrivels through lack of blood. Calcium salts may be deposited and these minute 'stones' are an extreme irritant and most likely to cause fits. In Sturge-Weber Syndrome there is an associated abnormality of the blood vessels of a part of the face giving a characteristic 'port-wine' stain. Although this is not very common, it is important since the blood vessel abnormality of the brain sometimes can be treated by operation.

b. Large arteries ramify over the surface of the brain before they send off branches to supply its substance. They lie under one of the coverings (meninges) which, because it is thin and whispy like a spider's web, is called the arachnoid. These blood vessels have little support and, if there is a weakness in the vessel wall, they are liable to rupture causing a disastrous and often fatal *subarachnoid haemorrhage*. If the patient survives, the free blood lying on the surface of the brain later acts as an extreme irritant liable to cause seizures. Since subarachnoid haemorrhages are due to a local weakness of the blood vessel, with which the patient is born, they often occur in young adults.

c. Older patients are liable to 'strokes' which are sudden catastrophies due to haemorrhage when a blood vessel bursts (often in those with high blood pressure): *thrombosis* when a vessel becomes blocked and the brain which it supplies is starved of blood and dies; or *embolism* when little blood clots formed elsewhere in the body become stuck in a brain blood vessel and again cause sudden loss of blood supply. Strokes may be fatal and, unless very slight, may cause loss of function such as paralysis or loss of sensation. If there is recovery, the resultant brain damage may give rise to seizures.

d. As people become older the brain blood vessels often become furred up or narrowed. The process is much more gradual than a stroke but nonetheless it results in death of small areas of brain. This causes the progressive mental changes found in many old people and it is also the most important cause of epilepsy in the old. Fortunately, the resulting seizures are usually mild and the epilepsy, which is not too difficult to control, is less of a disability than the mental deterioration.

8. Loss of brain substance (atrophy)

Many cases of brain *atrophy* are due to failure of blood supply. However, in a number of older people the brain starts to shrivel up for no reason which is understood presently. In the very old, such shrivelling is probably a part of the general process of ageing. In either case seizures are common, but, as when loss of brain substance is due to blood vessel disease, they are not particularly severe and do not represent the main problem.

Epilepsy (that is fits due to primary brain disorder) is represented diagrammatically in Figure 1.10, in which congenital brain sensitivity is plotted against acquired brain damage. Epilepsy results when there is a sufficient combination of brain sensitivity and brain damage. Those who lie below the diagonal line do not have a combination adequate to cause epilepsy; those unfortunates above the line suffer from epilepsy. Although the diagram is an over-simplification, it is useful in two ways. Firstly, it demonstrates the wide range of the population of people with epilepsy. Secondly, it is useful propaganda to dispel the concept of 'epileptics' as a group apart: people not quite like ourselves. Consider the effect of a particular degree of brain damage—as at X. Let us say that a roof collapsed on a group of people at a meeting and that each suffered an identical head injury with consequent brain damage. Those unfortunate enough to lie outwith the diagonal line, would later develop epilepsy, those under the line, would not. There is no us and them. We are all at risk.

Let us consider further the population of people with epilepsy represented in Figure 1.10. Brain damage affects the substance or structure of the brain: it is something which can be seen, if only under the microscope. Although there are occasions when the structural lesion can be removed at operation and the epilepsy alleviated or cured, it would not be expected that it would be influenced by changes in the environment. If therefore the brain damage cannot be altered by the environment, seizures due predominantly to the factor of brain damage would be less affected by environmental changes. Antiepileptic drugs act by effecting changes in the internal environment, and it is established that it is more difficult to control with drugs the fits of brain damaged patients. The effect of the external environment—the patient's reaction to what is going on round about him—is not so clear. The brain damaged patient with impaired intellect and emotional control is less competent to cope and so with adverse external circumstances more liable to behave inappropriately. The subsequent stress may act as a precipitant of fits. Nonetheless, the patient without brain damage, whose fits are due to brain sensitivity, may be liable to have his fits triggered by more subtle changes in his external circumstances.

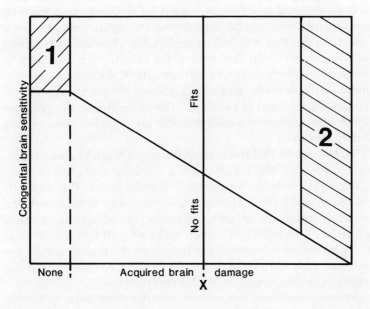

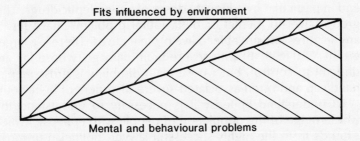

Fig. 1.10 A diagram to represent the population of people with epilepsy, as those with an adequate combination of the causative factors of congenital brain sensitivity and acquired brain damage. Those above the diagonal line have epilepsy, those below do not. The line drawn at X represents the same degree of brain damage. The lower part of the figure represents the relative influence of environment and the occurrence of mental and behavioural problems. The areas in the upper part marked 1 represent those whose epilepsy represents few problems, and 2 those whose main disability is mental handicap rather than epilepsy.

Brain sensitivity affects the way in which the brain works: it is a disorder of function. It cannot be demonstrated even by the electron microscope, although in the future it may be possible to show that it is influenced by the chemical substances which control brain function. Brain sensitivity is likely to be influenced by changes in environment. The external environment—stresses and strains—is known to effect changes in chemicals released in the brain. The antiepileptic drugs of the internal environment undoubtedly are capable of reducing brain sensitivity.

To the extent that the brain is damaged it is less able to function normally. The patient with a significant degree of brain damage is likely to be mentally handicapped. The mentally handicapped patient has an impaired ability to deal with the normal stresses to which he is subject. Unable to cope, he is more likely to react with severely disordered behaviour. Thus the greater the element of brain damage the greater will be the mental and behavioural problems of the patient whose epilepsy is due largely to such brain damage.

We may consider two extremes of the population of people with epilepsy. There is a comparatively small group (1) (Fig. 1.10) with no apparent brain damage; their seizures are able to be controlled well by regulation of the environment and in particular by adequate doses of antiepileptic drugs. This group have no mental or behavioural problems, have few if any seizures and are able to live ordinary lives. There is a larger group (2) (Fig. 1.10) with severe brain damage, whose fits are difficult to control, but whose main disability is gross mental handicap and often associated severe disorders of behaviour.

To understand epilepsy it is necessary to understand the whole range of the population of people with epilepsy. which extends from the highly successful lawyer, politician or musician (many examples are cited in the literature) to the convulsing village idiot, additionally handicapped by the stigmata of his mental handicap. For those whose job it is to help the person with epilepsy, it is so important to appreciate how wide is this range of population since so often the misfortunes of the latter group create misconceptions about the former.

2

Types of seizures

It is much easier to understand the different types of seizures with some knowledge of the structure and function of the nervous system. The description which follows has been simplified greatly. If such simplification offends the medical specialist (for whom this book is not written), there should be the compensation that it might interest rather than bore those for whom this book is written.

The nervous system effects rapid communication by means of the passage of minute electrical impulses and the release of chemical substances. It comprises millions upon millions of nerve cells. Each nerve cell consists of a nerve cell body, which organizes its working, and from which extend processes which receive (*dendrites*) and long fibres which transmit (*axons*) instructions. Some of the largest nerve cells have axons over a metre long (Fig. 2.1) and these are concerned—rather like telephone wires—with transmitting information to the brain or carrying instructions from it. Most nerve cells are microscopically small, grouped in very large inter-related masses, and concerned with collating and organizing information—they may be compared with a computer (Fig. 2.2).

The nervous system is usually divided into two parts. The central nervous system comprising the brain and the spinal

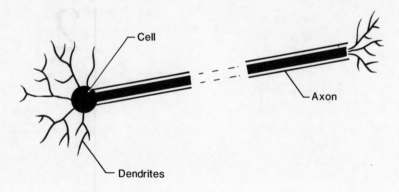

Fig. 2.1 Large nerve cell with long axon.

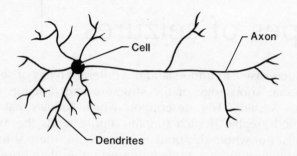

Fig. 2.2 Small nerve cell.

cord, which, because it is of particular importance, is protected by the skull and the bones of the spine. The peripheral nervous system consists of long nerve fibres which run from the skin, muscles and joints to carry information to the spinal cord, and others which carry instructions from the spinal cord to the muscles which control movements of the body and the functions of the internal organs. These peripheral nerves have less protection because, although damage to them causes loss of function, it does not threaten life. Peripheral nerves receiving information are called *sensory nerves*, those carrying instructions *motor nerves* (see Fig. 2.3).

The central nervous system is divided into *white matter* and *grey matter*. The long nerve fibres axons which carry messages are covered with a whitish fatty substance, which can be compared to the insulation on electric wires. Where axons are

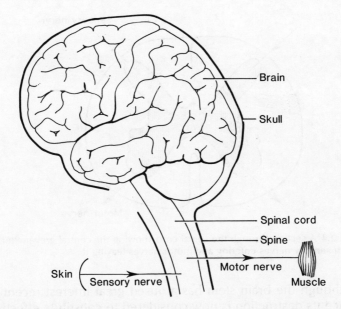

Fig. 2.3 The central nervous system consisting of the brain and spinal cord protected by the bony skull and spinal cord. The peripheral nervous system consisting of sensory nerves carrying information to and motor nerves instructions from the spinal cord.

grouped together the nervous tissue has a white appearance. Since the nerve cell bodies control the working of the nerves they need a much greater blood supply, and where they are grouped together they look darker or grey.

Much of the spinal cord consists of white matter, of the axons carrying messages to and from the brain. There is also a central core of grey matter where lie the cell bodies of the communication nerves and also many of the small computer-type nerves which ensure exchange of information and smooth working at a local level (Fig. 2.4). Seizures do not arise in the spinal cord and more detailed description is not necessary.

As the spinal cord extends upwards and enters the skull it is known as the brain stem. The brain stem consists largely of the white matter of communication axons, but with groups of grey matter comprising the cells controlling the muscles of the head, sensation from the head, and most importantly the vital functions of the body such as heart beat and respiration.

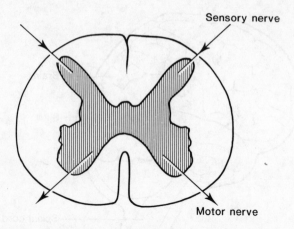

Fig. 2.4 A section through the spinal cord showing the central grey matter with sensory nerves entering and motor nerves leaving it.

Although the brain stem has aroused great interest recently, since its destruction is now considered to constitute effective death and so the occasion for shutting off life-support machines, like the spinal cord it is of no particular relevance to seizures, since few if any fits arise from it.

By far the greater part of the human brain consists of the *cerebral* hemispheres which sit—like conjoined cabbages—on the stalk of the brain stem. Discarding formal and complicated anatomical terminology, it is convenient to describe two zones: the Inner which consists of the upper part of the brain stem and the adjacent parts of the cerebral hemispheres; and the Outer, the bulk of the hemispheres. The Inner may be thought of as the older or more primitive since it is much the same in man as in other mammals. The Outer is the new brain in the sense that it is enormously developed in man and is much more important than in lower mammals.

The inner zone of the cerebral hemispheres and the upper brain stem.

This zone is immensely complicated and many of its functions are not yet understood fully. Through it pass the long axons running to and from the Outer Zone, but it consists mainly of enormous numbers of small nerve cells some of which are clustered together, whereas others are distributed in a network amidst the nerve fibres. It may be thought of as the main computer where incoming information is organized and related to appropriate outgoing instructions. It is of great importance to the understanding of epilepsy and we will consider some of its functions.

1. The long sensory axons carrying information up the spinal cord, not only relay before continuing to the Outer Zone, but also send numerous branches to the network of small cells. These are important in the maintenance of consciousness. It is possible for information to be relayed to the Outer Zone without a person being aware, or conscious, of what is happening. This happens during sleep when the consciousness part of the Inner Zone is resting, and when someone is unconscious as a result of serious illness, a severe head injury or an epileptic seizure.

2. The Inner Zone has important connections with a system of nerves (the *autonomic nervous system*), which controls the internal environment and the functions of internal organs: breathing control, the beating of the heart, movements of the gut, the bladder, the distribution of blood as between the skin and other parts of the body, and so on.

3. The nervous system is a rapid communications system, but there is also another slower system which controls internal workings: the endocrine system. This system releases chemical substances into the blood—hormones or endocrines. The control of the endocrine system lies in a small gland within the Inner Zone from which chemicals are released to exert long-term influence on such things as growth, sexual function, the rate at which the body works, the level of blood sugar, and the reaction to stress. While the nervous system influences the internal environment directly and quickly, it also influences this environment, indirectly and in the longer term, through its control of the endocrine system.

4. There is evidence that the Inner Zone is concerned with emotions such as fear, and with the emotional aspects of behaviour such as irritability and aggression.

5. Damage to certain parts within the Inner Zone are known to cause particular types of loss of memory (*amnesia*). Two aspects of memory need to be distinguished. Firstly, the

ability to record what is happening and lay it down as new memories: and secondly, the ability to make use of old memories which have already been laid down. The first is much more liable to be impaired. Without access to old memories, which include all that a person has learnt, it would be impossible for him to react appropriately to his environment. Therefore, someone who is behaving in a normal fashion must have access to memories of old experiences. The two aspects can be illustrated by the effects of a severe head injury. At first, the patient will be in a *coma* (completely unconscious). Thereafter, he will pass through a phase of confusion and partial consciousness until he becomes fully conscious and aware of his environment. He can go about his ordinary business behaving suitably and sensibly for several hours, but afterwards he will have complete amnesia for these hours (post-traumatic amnesia), because his brain has not recovered sufficiently to be able to store new memories of what has been happening.

6. The Inner Zone is closely connected to that part of the Outer Zone which receives information about taste and smell and to some extent sound. It is interesting that mammals more primitive than man depend more for their survival on these forms.

If, as we have suggested, the Inner Zone is involved in epileptic seizures, its manifold although improperly understood functions may explain some of the more complex features of the epileptic attack.

The outer zone of the cerebral hemispheres.

The cerebral hemispheres are covered with a mantle of nerve cells which forms a layer of grey matter, up to 4 mm thick, known as the *cortex*. Beneath the cortex the hemispheres consist of white matter: the axons of nerve cells which run from one part of the cortex to another, from one hemisphere to the other, from the cortex to the grey matter of the Inner Zone, and very long axons which run without relay to the grey matter of the brain stem and spinal cord*. Not only are the

---

* These long axons cross to the other side either in the brain stem or the spinal cord.

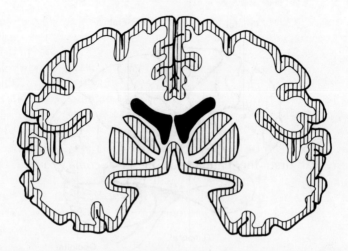

Fig. 2.5 A section through the cerebral hemispheres showing the grey matter of the cortex on the outside with other grey matter in central masses. The black central areas are the ventricles which contain fluid.

hemispheres in man much larger than in other mammals but they are thrown into numerous folds thus increasing very greatly the surface area of the cortex (Fig. 2.5).

The smaller folds (*sulci*) divide the surface into ridges termed *gyri* and deeper folds separate the hemispheres into *lobes* (Fig. 2.6). The greater part of the cortex forms a part of the computer system of the brain and has intimate communication through the axons of the white matter with the main computer system of the Inner Zone. However, certain surface areas have been shown to have more clearly defined functions. The gyrus behind the main central sulcus (*post-central* gyrus) receives sensory information from different parts of the body. If, for example, that part concerned with the mouth is stimulated electrically (and this may be done at operation to the conscious patient who will feel no pain since this part of the brain is not sensitive) the patient will have the sensation of tingling of the mouth. There is another area of the *occipital* lobe at the back of the brain concerned with receiving visual stimuli, and one where the temporal lobe adjoins the large lateral sulcus which receives sound stimuli. In front of the central sulcus is a strip of cortex (*pre-central* gyrus) which connects directly to the spinal cord and initiates movements;

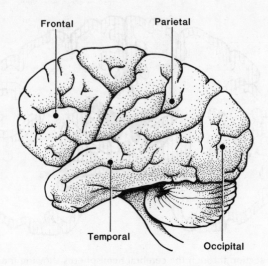

Frontal Parietal

Temporal

Occipital

Fig. 2.6 Side view of the left cerebral hemisphere showing the sulci and gyri with the division into frontal, parietal, temporal and occipital lobes.

for example, stimulation of the part controlling the thumb will cause the thumb to move. A little further forward there is another area concerned with movement of the head and eyes to one side, and near it one which is concerned with evoking speech (in right handed people speech is controlled from the left cerebral hemisphere).

Different parts of the precentral gyrus control movements in different parts of the body, from below upwards: tongue, mouth, face, thumb, fingers, hand, arm, trunk, leg with the foot and toes at the top in the dip between the two hemispheres. A disproportionate part of the gyrus is given over to those parts where fine movement control is necessary. Thus the tongue and lips, or the thumb and fingers, occupy a much larger area than the whole of the trunk. This body representation is reflected in the post-central gyrus which receives sensation from the body. Because the long axons cross (p. 26) the left pre-central gyrus controls the right side of the body and the left post-central gyrus receives sensation from the right (Fig. 2.7).

We have given some detail of the structure of the cerebral cortex because of its importance in the understanding of certain types of seizures. As far as is known, seizures originate in the nerve cell bodies of the grey matter, either of the cortex or within the Inner Zone. It should be noted that the inner parts of the temporal lobes, and to a lesser extent the deeper parts of the frontal lobes, merge with and form an important part of the Inner Zone.

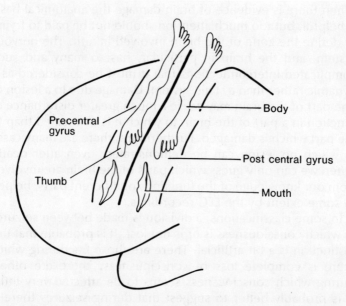

Fig. 2.7 A scheme of the left pre-central and post-central gyri showing the way in which the body is represented. Note the large area for the mouth and hand, particularly the thumb.

Seizures may be grouped or classified in three different ways:

a. In clinical terms, that is what an observer sees happening during an attack
b. In electrical terms, that is what is recorded on the electroencephalograph (EEG) (p. 32) while the attack is taking place
c. In anatomical terms, that is by describing the part of the brain in which the seizure is presumed to have started and the parts to which it has spread.

The official classifications are enormously complicated, constant attempts are being made to revise them, and although we will try to follow them we will make no attempt to describe them. In this chapter we will consider only the commonest types of seizures and we will base our grouping on the clinical features of the attack with reference to the EEG findings and use diagrams to suggest the anatomical basis. When there is evidence of brain damage the anatomical basis is helpful, but too much attention should not be paid to trying to define the zone of the brain involved in a fit. The nervous system, and the brain in particular, has so many and such complicated interconnections that it must be considered as a dynamic rather than a static system. Damage due to a lesion of one part of the brain may cause a much greater disturbance of function in a part of the brain to which it is connected than to the part which is damaged. Furthermore, there are many cases in which no lesion can be demonstrated, even after death. Often we can only guess which parts of the brain are involved from our knowledge of the functions of different parts, helped to some extent by the EEG recordings.

In some classifications, a division is made between seizures in which consciousness is or is not lost. It is probable that this distinction is a bit artificial. There are those fits during which there is complete loss of consciousness: there are others during which consciousness seems to be affected very little. It is probably better to suggest that during seizures there is a very wide range of alteration of consciousness: from complete loss to a state in which alteration is difficult to detect. It is useful to define consciousness as an awareness of environment combined with the ability to react appropriately. There are certain slight (or partial) seizures, which we will describe, during which the patient appears to be fully conscious but when he is unable to control either involuntary movements or the appreciation of abnormal sensations.

We have suggested that the masses of computer-type nerve cells in the Inner Zone are important to consciousness. This Inner network has intimate connections with nerve cells of the cortex which also have a computer function and so are concerned to some extent with what we have described as consciousness. We suggest that the degree to which consciousness is impaired depends on the extent of the disturbance of function of the computer-type cells wherever they may be.

In the first instance we can divide seizures into three groups:

1. Primary generalized seizures in which:
   a. Consciousness is lost from the beginning
   b. There is EEG evidence of disturbance affecting all those parts from which the EEG can be recorded
   c. No evidence can be found of a lesion responsible for the seizure.
2. Partial seizures in which:
   a. There is no immediate loss of consciousness, and in some cases any loss of consciousness may be very slight
   b. It may be possible to record a local EEG disturbance
   c. There is presumed to be a causative lesion although this may be difficult to detect.
3. Secondary generalized seizures.

These develop from the spread of partial seizures. Some people have partial seizures which never become generalized. Others have partial seizures which may or may not spread. Clearly, brain damage plays an important part in the production of partial attacks, and it seems reasonable to suggest that the tendency to spread is a measure of brain sensitivity. In those cases when partial seizures only rarely become generalized it may be that such occasional spread is triggered by some factor outside the brain—some change in the internal environment.

Primary generalized seizures

1. Simple absences (petit mal)

Although it is quite correct to talk of *petit mal absences*, the term petit mal is liable to cause confusion since many people use it to describe any slight attack.

These are the slightest of attacks and are almost limited to children. The child loses consciousness, quite suddenly, for about ten seconds. He does not fall and makes no movements apart from perhaps brief muscle twitches or eye blinks. He recovers equally suddenly, appears a little surprised at what has happened, but then carries on with what he was doing. Some children have hundreds of these absences in a day and in such cases they may interfere seriously with school

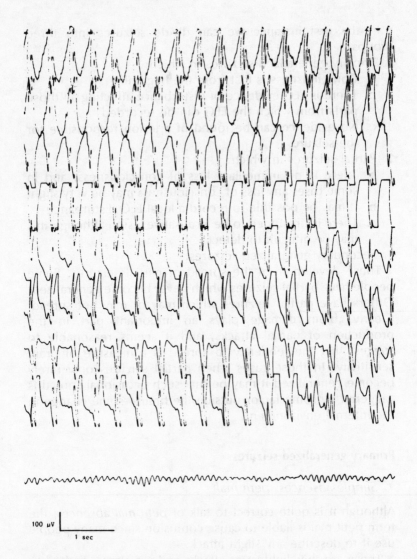

100 μV

1 sec

Fig. 2.8 A simple absence in a child. See also legend for 1.1.

work. Sometimes, they also have occasional jerking of the muscles (*myoclonus*) and, much less commonly, attacks in which their muscles relax suddenly and they fall, only to recover immediately. Almost all cases of simple absences start before adolescence and the great majority stop by the age of about 20. Some children later develop *tonic-clonic convulsions* (see below).

During the attack there is a very characteristic electrical disturbance which can be shown on the EEG (see Fig. 2.8 and p. 6 for explanation). It is usually suggested that simple absences arise in the network of cells at the centre of the Inner Zone. However, there must be some involvement of the cortex since the EEG measures the electrical activity of the cortex. Nevertheless, it is convenient to represent a simple absence, as in Figure 2.9, where there is a brain free of brain damage with a deeply placed disturbance.

A simple absence is a true example of a primary generalized seizure. No other type of seizure develops from a simple absence. There is no brain damage and the attack may be thought of as due entirely to brain sensitivity. Because there is no brain damage the child will be quite normal mentally, although if the attacks are very frequent he may have learning difficulties. It is interesting that this type of seizure is particularly sensitive to the changes in the internal environment produced by overbreathing.*

This type of attack is not very common, although the percentages quoted are possibly an underestimate since some patients may not be referred, for what are slight seizures, to the neurological centres which produce statistics.

2. Tonic-clonic convulsions (grand mal).

The grand mal fit is the most dramatic and frightening of all seizures. It is not surprising that most people, when they think of epilepsy, think of a tonic-clonic convulsion. In fact the primary type is quite easy to treat and should be rare.

Suddenly, without warning, there is a contraction of the muscles (the *tonic phase*). Often the patient lets out a wild cry. He loses consciousness at once, and always falls. Then, for up to two minutes his muscles alternately relax and contract again (the *clonic phase*). A great deal of saliva is produced and with the strong contractions of his chest

---

* Overbreathing washes carbon dioxide out of the blood. Carbon dioxide controls the diameter of the blood vessels of the brain. When the level is low the vessels contract and less blood and hence less oxygen gets to the brain.

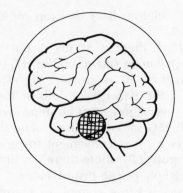

Fig. 2.9 Simple absence.

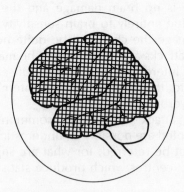

Fig. 2.10 Primary tonic-clonic convulsion.

muscles this will be forced out of his mouth as a froth. If, as quite often happens, the contractions of the jaw muscles have caused him to bite his tongue or cheek, the froth will be blood stained. The awesome picture is compounded by contortions of the facial muscles which render the familiar face terrifyingly unrecognizable. Normal breathing is impossible, the blood becomes short of oxygen and the contorted face becomes blue or almost black (*cyanosis*). The pupils dilate and the patient sweats profusely. If there is an appreciable amount of urine in the bladder, the contractions will cause water to be passed. Less often he soils himself (is *incontinent* of faeces).

Gradually the clonic contractions become less strong and less frequent until with a final jerk or two he falls into a state

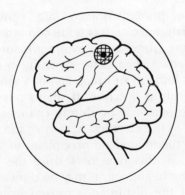

Fig. 2.11 Simple partial seizure.

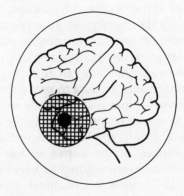

Fig. 2.12 Complex partial seizure.

of deep unconsciousness (coma) from which he cannot be roused. This stage usually lasts about five minutes—although it may be considerably longer. Slowly he recovers but he will be in a state of altered consciousness and will be confused. It is important to appreciate that he is not aware fully of what is happening. If he is interfered with, he may lash out wildly in his confusion. He is not violent or dangerous, merely unable to react appropriately to a situation which he is not sufficiently conscious to appreciate. On recovery, he usually has a headache and his muscles feel bruised and sore.

There may be variations to the full-blown seizure, particularly after treatment and in infants and young children. There may be only a tonic or only a clonic phase.

Although the primary tonic-clonic convulsion occurs without immediate warning it is quite common for patients to have rather vague (*prodromal*) symptoms for hours or even days before an attack: headache, difficulty in sleeping, mood changes such as lethargy or irritability, or a sense of tenseness which it is difficult to describe. It seems possible that these prodromal symptoms may be due to changes in the internal environment or in the electrical activity of the brain, which in turn may act as the immediate precipitant of the seizure.

By definition, in this type of seizure the whole brain is involved from the beginning. It may be difficult to record the EEG because of the disturbance caused by movement and muscle contractions (see *artefacts*, p. 69) but, in as far as the electrical changes in the brain can be shown, there is nothing to suggest that they start locally. Because consciousness is lost at the very beginning there is no warning (*aura*) to suggest that the attack has started in any particular part of the brain.

There are, however, difficulties in adducing either the EEG findings or the absence of an aura to prove that a tonic-clonic convulsion is primary—that is due wholly to brain sensitivity and not at all to some lesion, some brain damage, which initiates the attack. Firstly, the EEG is recorded only from the exposed outer surface of the cortex of the cerebral hemispheres. An electrical event starting in some deep area inaccessible to the EEG might be manifest only when it had become generalized to involve the surface cortex from which the EEG can be recorded. Secondly, while there are areas of the brain in which disturbance results in clinically apparent change, there are large parts of the computer-type brain which are clinically silent. A lesion in these areas might initiate a convulsion without apparent warning.

At one time it was thought that primary grand mal epilepsy was quite common. Increasingly improved methods of investigation have been able to show the presence of more and more previously hidden provocative lesions: that more and more tonic-clonic convulsions are secondary.

Although there are those who would contend that there is no such thing as a primary tonic-clonic convulsion, this is probably an extreme view. It would seem more likely that this form of seizure is comparatively rare but that there is a small number of people liable to such seizures because of a degree of brain sensitivity adequate to cause fits without the additional factor of a brain lesion. This group would be comparable to those with simple absences and might include those with simple absences who later develop grand mal. In either case these patients are fortunate in that the fits are able to be controlled more easily and that in the absence of brain damage they are not at risk of primary disturbance of intellect or behaviour. This group may be represented by Figure 2.10. In the absence of a brain lesion there is a sudden explosive electrical disturbance involving the grey matter of the Inner Zone and of the cortex. The areas of cortex controlling movements send meaningless instructions which causes widespread contraction of muscles.

Partial seizures

Partial seizures involve a disturbance in a localized zone of the brain. They may be presumed to be due to a brain lesion, ranging from a slight scar the result of old damage, to an actively developing tumour. Unless the lesion is situated in a part inaccessible to the surface, it is often possible to record a localized change on the EEG. Unless the disturbance spreads widely, there is not loss of consciousness, although there is some degree of alteration of consciousness.

Partial seizures may be either simple or complex. Simple when a part of the brain concerned with simple functions is involved, and complex when more complex functions are affected. In the simple type, little of what we have termed the computer brain is affected and there may be hardly any detectable alteration of consciousness. Complex partial seizures involve an appreciable alteration of consciousness since they affect the Inner Zone and its connections with the deeper parts of the temporal or frontal lobes.

1. Simple partial seizures

These arise in or spread quickly to those parts of the cortex described on page 28 and shown in Figure 2.7. Thus, arising in the thumb area of the pre-central gyrus the attack would start with jerking movements of the thumb, perhaps spreading to the fingers and with involvement of the adjoining post-central gyrus causing numbness of, or pins and needles in, the hand. Such attacks are often quite limited but they may spread through the pre-central gyrus: downwards to the face and upwards to the arm trunk and leg. With extensive spread there will be loss of consciousness and a secondary tonic-clonic seizure, probably involving particularly the side first affected*. Other simple partial seizures may start in the post-central gyrus with, say, numbness of the lips; in the visual area of the occipital lobe with simple sensations such as flashing lights; or in that part of the frontal lobe controlling movements of the head and eyes, when the head and eyes will turn to the opposite side.

After seizures which have involved extensive and persistent movements of one side of the body it is common for there to be weakness of this side for some hours. A patient should be reassured that such temporary weakness is not something to be alarmed about. However, should it persist for more than, say, 24 hours, it should be reported to the doctor since it may indicate the presence of a tumour or the occurrence of a stroke.

A simple partial seizure is represented in Figure 2.11 in which the circle suggests the zone involved and the black area the causative lesion.

2. Complex partial seizures

It used to be thought that this group of seizures always originated in the temporal lobe, and therefore it was referred to as temporal lobe epilepsy. It is now known that occasionally attacks may start in adjacent zones and so the term complex partial seizures is more suitable.

The types of seizures which we have described so far, each form a fairly homogeneous group subject to only minor variations. By contrast complex partial seizures, because of the involvement of a part of the brain with a wide variety of different functions, form an extremely heterogeneous group, varying not only in severity, depending on the extent of the brain concerned, but also in their manifestation according to

---

* These seizures are more likely to start in a part of the body having a large area of representation on the pre-central gyrus—e.g. lips, tongue or thumb.

the parts of the brain concerned. Some of the functions of the Inner Zone have been described (p. 25). Let us consider further different elements, various of which combine to form a particular complex partial seizure, but which will tend to be more or less the same for any individual patient.

a. Actions. The pre-central gyrus controls the contractions of muscles and muscle groups. The movements of a simple partial seizure (p. 37) are, therefore, simple and quite purposeless—jerking of the thumb or arm, twitching of the mouth. The computer brain of the Inner Zone organizes muscular contractions to a programme of purposive actions appropriate to the external environment of which the computer is aware because of the sensory information which is being fed into it. During a seizure movements will still be organized into actions but, because a seizure is an abnormal event, the actions will be abnormal and to a degree inappropriate. They are referred to as semipurposive movements or automatisms. These automatisms may occur during the seizure itself, or, more often, during the period of confusion which follows. They vary in complexity. In the simpler, the patient may smack his lips, make chewing movements, or fiddle with his clothes. In the more complex, which are more likely to follow an attack, he may start to undress, or, say, wander about the room picking up objects and putting them down in the wrong place. Automatisms seldom last longer than a few minutes although amnesia following a complex seizure may last longer (p. 42). Disturbed behaviour which goes on for hours cannot be attributed to epilepsy and it is usually possible to show that it has been carried out in clear consciousness, that is to say it bears a meaningful relationship to the environment. The medico-legal importance of such behaviour will be considered later (p. 138–139).

b. Sensory information. Areas of the cerebral cortex which receive simple sensations have been described (see p. 27)—touch from the body, sight or sound from the eyes or from the ears. It is only when these sensations are organized by the computer brain and are appreciated by a conscious person that they have meaning. A simple partial (sensory) seizure involving the occipital lobe might consist of flashing lights (p. 38). The sensory component of a complex partial seizure is more meaningful, but because it is due to abnormal brain activity, it is only semi-meaningful—an hallucination, which is unrelated to what is actually happening in the external environment. For example, at the beginning of his attack a patient may see seagulls wheeling over a rocky coast and hear the thunder of the sea in the background. Perhaps this is a reactivation of old memory traces stored in the computer brain.

The deeper parts of the temporal lobe accept the primitively important sensations of taste and smell. Quite often at the start of a complex partial seizure a patient will appreciate a taste or a smell. For some reason, perhaps because the sensation is due to abnormal activity, it is nearly always unpleasant and described as foul, horrible, obscene or just indescribable.

The ear is concerned not only with hearing but also with balance and the appreciation of position in space. Information from the ear is received in the temporal lobe, and it is common for a complex partial seizure to be heralded by a sensation of dizziness.

c. Autonomic effects. The deeper parts of the temporal and frontal lobes have close connections with the autonomic nerves which receive information from the internal organs (of which we are not usually aware) and organize the working of the body in a way over which we have no conscious control.

During the early part of a complex partial seizure, before consciousness is affected much, the patient may be aware of bodily sensations, which, because they are due to brain disturbance rather than impulses from the organ involved, are often difficult to describe. For example: 'Before one of my turns I have a weird feeling in my stomach which spreads to my chest and throat. I feel as if I am suffocating and being strangled. It is horrible.' Such an early sensation provides a warning (aura) that a seizure is coming on.

During a complex partial seizure inappropriate instructions may be transmitted by the autonomic nerves resulting in disturbed body function, which may be embarrassing: sweating, flushing or pallor of the skin, alterations in breathing, changes in heart rate, excessive bowel movement which may cause very loud borborygmi (tummy rumbles) and the passing of wind. The patient is often incontinent and this is more probably an autonomic effect than the incontinence due to the generalized muscles contractions which occur during a tonic-clonic convulsion.

d. Disturbance of thought, perception and emotion. Since the masses of nerve cells of the Inner Zone are involved, it might be expected that the patient would have psychological experiences, as long as a degree of consciousness was retained adequate for him to appreciate them. However, in as far as there is likely to be a degree of alteration of consciousness, this appreciation will be impaired and the experiences difficult to describe and often bizarre.

Quite commonly a patient will have an overwhelming feeling that the events which are occurring around him—in his external environment—have all happened before (*déjà vu*). The word overwhelming is important since many ordinary people, who are not having seizures, have from time to time a vague sense of familiarity. Much less commonly he may have the feeling that familiar objects around him are strange and unreal (*jamais vu*).

Occasionally perception may be distorted. A patient's body may seem enormous or minute in relation to his environment, or external events may seem to be happening very very slowly, like an action replay of a sporting event.

It is common for appreciation of the early part of a complex partial seizure to be associated with a pervading emotion. Such emotions are almost always unpleasant, the most usual being fear, or the minor fear that is severe anxiety. The emotional experience, of which the patient is likely to have only a brief memory, may be detached from any other sensory experience—'I was overcome with a sudden feeling of terror, but I cannot describe by what I was terrified'. Alternatively the emotion may be associated with another sensory experience—'I had this feeling of oppression in my chest and an acute anxiety that I was going to die'. Despite the often quoted ecstatic experiences of Dostoevski's Prince Myshkin in *The Idiot*, pleasant emotions are most uncommon. Rarely, there may be an associated erotic experience. Rage and anger do not seem to play a part in complex seizures and if a patient appears to be violent or dangerous this is not a part of his attack but much more probably the confused reaction to well meaning interference when he is only partially conscious during recovery.

These psychological experiences form the early part or aura of the seizure. It is often difficult to get a clear description from the patient since, like a dream, they arise when there is some alteration of consciousness, and being abnormal experiences it is difficult to describe them in everyday terms.

e. Memory. The complex hallucinations which initiate a patient's seizure (p. 40) may, like a dream, be a composite playback of old memories. Some patients have a period after apparent full recovery, which may be compared to post-traumatic amnesia (p. 16). They react to their environment in a perfectly normal manner but they have no recollection afterwards of this period. It may be assumed that those parts of the brain concerned with registering new memories have been exhausted by the seizure; a situation similar to weakness after a motor attack (p. 38).

f. Consciousness. Because of the intimate relationship to central grey matter, in contrast to simple partial seizures the complex seizures involve a greater alteration of consciousness. There are two points of interest.

Of the various components of the seizure, alteration of consciousness may predominate with few other manifestations. Such attacks may mimic the simple absences, which we have described. They may be referred to as *complex absences*. It is important to distinguish between them, since both the treatment and the patient's future prospects (*prognosis*) are different. Complex absences last longer, are usually associated with some other features of the complex partial seizure such as slight semi-purposive movements—lip-smacking or fumbling—, and they do not have the sudden switch-on and switch-off of the simple absence.

Mrs W lived with her sister Mrs Y in a respectable suburb of a large city. They had much in common including their widowhood. Mrs W suffered from epilepsy, but only occasionally did this disturb the settled regularity of their lives.

However, at first their happily adjusted relationship nearly foundered on the rocks of Mrs W's epilepsy. Mrs Y could not understand why her usually easy natured sister unpredictably should be so frankly unkind, even rude. Perhaps their decision to live together had been a disaster. However, money was tight and Mrs Y could not move out until she had time to make new plans. The delay was fortunate since she came to realise that her sister's uncharacteristic and hurtful behaviour was related to her fits.

Mrs Y began to watch her sister more closely. When other people were present she seemed to fade out of the conversation. She became inaccessible, her face paled then her lips seemed to be blue and she starting making chewing movements. Soon her normal colour returned but she would start to fumble clumsily with her clothes or anything else to hand. If she had been knitting, she would get into a terrible mess. These episodes would last only two or three minutes, but for at least 20 minutes she would be different: she would be irritable and abrasive. Back to her usual self, she would have no memory of what had happened.

Comment

Mrs W had been having complex partial seizures with alteration of consciousness. She was in no way responsible for her behaviour. It must have been difficult for Mrs Y to understand what had been happening, but once she did appreciate the bizarre nature of her fits, the two widows lived happily ever after. The odd 20 minutes, now and again, could be ignored —just one of those things.

We have suggested (p. 37) that a primary tonic-clonic seizure is due to an explosive electrical disturbance involving the grey matter of both the Inner Zone and the cortex. Because of the involvement of the Inner Zone in a complex partial seizure, this type of fit is especially liable to spread to the cortex and result in a secondary tonic-clonic seizure. In many cases this spread is so rapid that the early stages of the complex partial seizure are not immediately apparent. In fact the great majority of tonic-clonic seizures are not primary but are secondary to a complex partial one. Whenever there is an aura, the seizure is not primary, and most aurae represent those early parts of a partial seizure which we have described and which are remembered by the patient because consciousness was not lost fully.

A complex partial seizure may be represented in Figure 2.12.

Secondary generalized seizures

The development of secondary generalized seizures may be represented in Figure 2.13. Of generalized seizures: the simple absence is never secondary to a partial seizure, nor is the primary tonic-clonic convulsion although this type of seizure is rare and is clinically indistinguishable from a secondary tonic-clonic seizure. Partial seizures may or may not

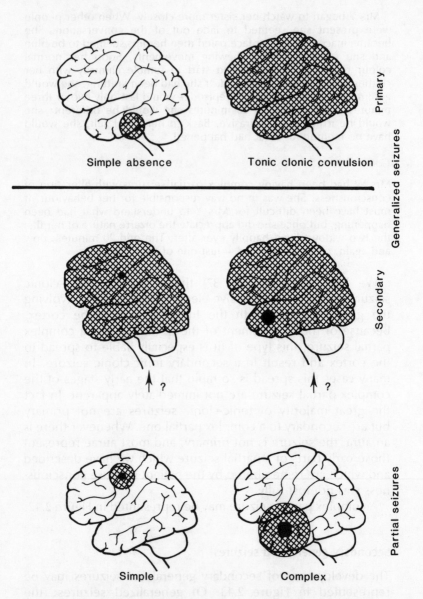

Simple absence   Tonic clonic convulsion

Primary

Generalized seizures

Secondary

?   ?

Simple   Complex

Partial seizures

Fig. 2.13 As for Figs. 2.9. to 2.12. Simple and complex partial seizures may develop to give secondary generalized seizures. Note the absence of brain damage in the primary generalized seizures—simple absence and tonic-clonic convulsion—which do not develop from any other type of fit.

develop; if they do, whether simple or complex, they result in a similar type of tonic-clonic fit.

Although not a part of the classification of seizures, two seizure events should be described in this chapter.

Status epilepticus

This is the condition when a number of seizures—of whatever type occur without recovery of consciousness in between. The term *serial seizures* is used when there is return to consciousness between attacks. Often serial fits are a warning that *status epilepticus* is impending.

1. Tonic-clonic convulsions. This type of status (epilepticus) constitutes a medical emergency. The great majority of tonic-clonic convulsions are self-limiting. The convulsing brain becomes exhausted, is unable to convulse any more, and the patient will sink into a coma from which he will recover. For some reason, in status each seizure seems to make the brain more liable to another. If status continues for many hours the resultant changes in the internal environment are so severe that the patient dies. Short of death the brain may suffer significant permanent damage. However, the danger of brain damage should not be exaggerated. Even status lasting for as short a time as an hour may cause brain damage to the immature brain of the young child (see febrile convulsions p. 152), and elegant experiments on baboons have demonstrated resultant damage from induced status. This does not mean that status in adults, vigorously and effectively treated, need necessarily have such long-term consequences: rather it emphasizes the importance of emergency treatment.

Unlike the apparently random occurrence of the great majority of ordinary tonic-clonic convulsions, it is often possible to show a precipitant cause for status epilepticus. In many cases status is the first manifestation of epilepsy due to brain damage—meningitis, a vascular accident or a brain tumour. After the status has been controlled it is, of course, mandatory to carry out the appropriate investigations to find the cause. When patients with known epilepsy develop status there is usually an apparent cause. Perhaps there has been a sudden reduction in antiepileptic drugs, whether ordered by the doctor or because the patient has decided to change his treatment or failed to observe it. Perhaps he has some infection which has disturbed his internal environment. If there is no such apparent precipitant, it is often important that he should be investigated further to exclude some potentially remediable cause. If a patient is considered to be having excessive doses of antiepileptic drugs, and it is necessary to reduce these drugs, it is often wise that such a reduction should be carried out in a hospital or an Epilepsy Centre, when any possible status can be dealt with quickly.

'Status' has been described in other types of seizure, although, since there is not continuing loss of consciousness, the term 'serial' would be more strictly correct, and also contrasted with true status epilepticus there is not the same danger to life or of brain damage.

2. Absences. Children may have very frequently repeated absence attacks which can continue for hours or days. In the past such serial attacks have been missed and the child has been described as 'day-dreaming' or 'difficult'. These serial absences can be picked up if the child is observed carefully. There are usually slight clues such as eye blinks or slight muscle twitches (myoclonus). However, this is one of the situations when the EEG can make a definitive diagnosis. Although not as rare as they were once thought to be, serial absences do not account for all children whom teachers find inattentive or tiresome! Nevertheless, it is important that teachers should be aware of the possibility so that doubtful cases are referred to the School Medical Officer, or, through the parents, to the GP.

3. Complex partial seizures. Rather rarely these also may be serial and again the diagnosis can be confirmed by the EEG. The patient will behave for long periods in an inappropriate fashion and he will have no subsequent recollection of what has happened (amnesia). These states last longer than the automatisms or periods of exhaustion amnesia which we have described as following a complex seizure. In the latter the EEG does not show the electrical discharges characteristic of continuing epileptic activity.

4. Simple partial seizures. Rather rarely a simple partial seizure may continue, without spread and therefore with little alteration of consciousness, for days or even weeks. The twitching contractions usually involve either the mouth or the hand (p. 38). This condition goes under the somewhat formidable name of 'epilepsia partialis continua'. It would seem that there is little brain sensitivity, and so little tendency to spread, but a high degree of provocative brain damage. Most cases are due to a localized head injury or a small stroke (vascular accident). If these causes can be excluded, it is important to carry out tests to make sure that the patient does not have a brain tumour.

Febrile convulsions *(see also p. 152)*

It is quite common for children between the ages of six months and five years (more than half between 9 and 20 months) to have convulsions when they have an infection which causes a high temperature. In most cases such convulsions are harmless in the sense that they cause no brain damage and so do not imply any risk of the development of recurrent fits (epilepsy) in later life. In general, the seizures are similar to the tonic-clonic convulsions which we have described but they may be atypical and involve only one side of the body. Because they are so common they are of especial importance. The parents will need reassurance, and there are circumstances in which they may cause damage to the temporal lobes and, thus, later complex partial seizures. It is essential that parents should be aware of these circumstances so that they can take appropriate action to prevent later epilepsy.

3

The patient and
the doctor

Disorders* have a natural history. An acute infection is only very rarely fatal; in nearly every case it clears up with or without suitable treatment. Cancers, although they can be treated effectively, all too often show a progressive decline to death. Multiple sclerosis, for which there is presently no known treatment, follows a long course, perhaps interrupted by long periods of relative freedom, but usually resulting in increasing disability. And so on.

Epilepsy is a disorder the diagnosis of which carries far too great an implication of impending doom. Figure 3.1 attempts firstly to put the disorder into proper perspective—to remove nearly all the doom, and secondly, to form a basis for the discussion in this chapter of the various stages of the patient's relationship to his doctors. The figure is meant to be illustrative rather than numerically accurate and it excludes that quite large number of patients with severe brain damage and consequent mental handicap, whose problem is mental handicap rather than epilepsy, and who are looked after by doctors concerned with the greater disability.

---

* The word disorder is used since epilepsy should not be thought of as a disease or even necessarily as a disability.

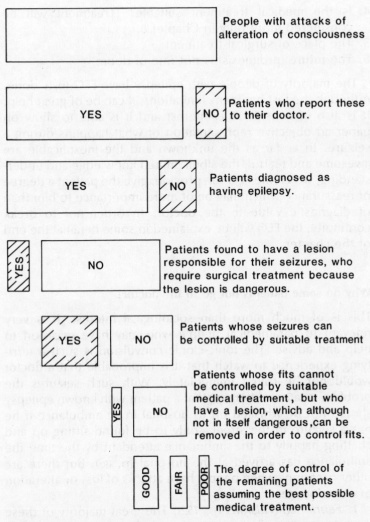

Fig. 3.1 A representation of the various stages through which a population of people with attacks of loss of consciousness (upper block) pass, until a small number are left with continuing seizures (three lower blocks).

This chapter is divided into the six sections shown in Figure 3.1.

1. Why do some patients not go to the doctor?
2. Is the attack epilepsy?
3. Investigations to try to find a cause for the epilepsy.

4. Is the medical treatment suitable? (Treatment will be considered more fully in Chapter 8.)
5. The place of surgical treatment.
6. The future (prognosis) is not one of doom.

The majority of people with epilepsy have EEG tests done. Although the test has many limitations, it can be of great help. It is also of considerable interest and it is able to show on paper an objective representation of what happens during a seizure. In as far as the unknown and the inexplicable are awesome and fearful, the albeit limited knowledge and understanding, which the EEG can provide, give the patient a degree of reassurance which may be of more importance to him than of diagnostic value to the doctor. In order not to break continuity, the EEG will be explained in some detail at the end of the chapter.

Why do some patients not go to the doctor?

This is of much more than sociological interest. It is very relevant to paramedical people who may have occasion to help and advise. The tonic-clonic convulsion is such a terrifying experience to watch that it is improbable that a doctor would not be called immediately. With such seizures the problem is rather different: that a patient with known epilepsy should not be whisked off to hospital in an ambulance if he has a seizure in the street—only to be found sitting up and chatting happily to the ambulance attendant by the time the ambulance has arrived at the hospital (p. 86). But there are other occasions when people have attacks of loss or alteration of consciousness.

1. Febrile convulsions (p. 152). The great majority of these are of no serious importance and do not result in later epilepsy. The mother may have the impression from neighbours' hearsay that they are just 'one of those things': to be accepted as a part of a child's growing up. Although in many cases this is so, it is essential that a doctor should be called, since there are occasions when a febrile convulsion is more serious.

2. Other causes of loss of consciousness. These will be considered in the next section and the district nurse, social worker, or teacher should have an understanding of events such as simple faints in order to be able to reassure the patient and his family. However, if there is any doubt at all, it is better to be on the safe side and get a medical opinion.

3. Fear. We are all afraid of being ill. As we have said, the diagnosis of epilepsy carries with it the quite unnecessary diagnosis of doom. There are quite a few people who will not approach a doctor for fear of hearing the truth. The paramedical worker can do a great deal to impress the importance of visiting the doctor, and can explain that even if the dread diagnosis is made, it is not necessarily so dreadful, and in any event correct diagnosis and proper treatment is essential to make it less so

4. Simple absences. Although these are less common than used to be thought, they are liable to be missed. Paramedicals, and particularly teachers, are often able to advise parents or School Medical Officers that reference should be made for a definitive diagnosis of apparent vagueness. The points described in Chapter 2 will help to avoid unnecessary referrals.

5. Complex partial seizures. Some of these do not develop to secondary tonic-clonic convulsions and so their significance may be missed or misinterpreted. Since they are notoriously difficult to control with antiepileptic drugs, it might be argued that no great harm would be done unless or until a major fit supervened. There is force in this argument since many attacks, which are not complex partial seizures, have been treated wrongly as such and have resulted in the unnecessary classification of a person as suffering from epilepsy. However, there are two caveats.

a. These strange attacks often cause great anxiety to patients, since, because they do not understand them, they feel that they are going 'odd' or even 'mad.' Such anxieties should be resolved by the doctor.

b. In older patients some of these more bizarre attacks may be the first sign of a brain tumour. Although this is not often the case, only medical reference can exclude the possibility.

Is the attack epilepsy?

Although medical books list a large number of disorders which may be confused with epilepsy, many of these are rare and require special medical tests. We will mention these for their general interest and in as far as patients may want to know what the tests are all about.

Most alternative diagnoses (*differential diagnosis*) are quite easily appreciated without specialist medical training although sometimes doctors with special experience need to make the final decision. Since it is unusual for a doctor to witness the attack, he is very dependent on the account (history) which he is given. Therefore, it is important to consider these common conditions fully so that observers know what to report.

In Chapter 1 we considered conditions outside the brain which might cause fits. Some of these conditions, which do not go as far as to cause convulsions, nevertheless so impair the function of the brain that there is a loss or alteration of consciousness which will need to be distinguished from epilepsy. Psychological disturbances may result in episodic behaviour disorders which may be difficult to distinguish from complex partial seizures.

The characteristics of most epileptic attacks are shown in Figure 3.2. They start and stop suddenly and there is seldom an apparent immediate precipitant.

1. Failure of the quantity or quality of the blood reaching the brain.

a. Faints (syncope). In the simple and common faint there is a disturbance of the distribution of blood through the body (controlled by the autonomic nervous system p. 25) so that the brain does not get enough. Blood accumulates in the lower parts of the body, the heart slows and the blood pressure falls. The onset is gradual, there is a feeling of dizziness or a sinking feeling. The patient will become pale, may sweat, and will fall in a gradual way, crumpling up, and so will seldom hurt himself. As soon as he is horizontal blood will flow back to his brain and he will recover fairly quickly but will feel nauseated. A faint can be distinguished from an epileptic seizure in two main ways (Fig. 3.3):

(i) Both the onset and the recovery are more gradual.

(ii) There is some apparent precipitant. Blood may accumulate in the lower limbs if someone has been standing for a long time without moving, as happens to a soldier on

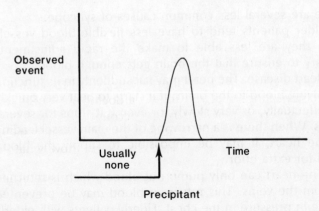

Fig. 3.2 Time scale of an epileptic seizure which starts and stops suddenly and for which there is usually no precipitant.

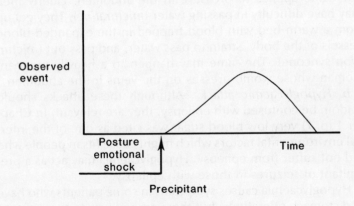

Fig. 3.3 Time scale of a simple faint with gradual onset and recovery and which is precipitated by emotional shock or change of posture.

parade, or, in a warm atmosphere, blood vessels will expand, and, if someone gets up suddenly, adjustments are not made quickly enough to ensure adequate blood being redistributed to the brain. Alternatively, a sudden emotional shock such as an injection or the sight of blood will upset the autonomic nervous system and cause a fall in blood pressure and slowing of the heart.

Simple faints usually affect young people, and more often young women.

There are several less common causes of syncope.

(i) Older patients tend to have less flexible blood vessels and so they are less able to make the rapid adjustments necessary to ensure that the brain gets enough blood.

(ii) Heart disease. The heart may fail suddenly in its function of supplying blood to the brain: if it starts to beat very quickly and ineffectually, or very slowly, or even if it stops for several seconds. When there is a narrowing of the main vessel leading from the heart, it may be impossible to supply the blood needed for extra effort.

(iii) The heart can only pump out blood which is returned to it from the veins. This return of blood may be prevented by a rise in pressure in the chest. Elderly patients with elderly blood vessels, often men with chest trouble, may precipitate syncope by a prolonged spasm of coughing (cough syncope). The same applies to pressure in the abdomen. Elderly men may have difficulty in passing water (*micturating*). They get up from a warm bed with blood trapped in the expanded blood vessels of the body, strain to pass water, and pass out (*micturition* syncope). The same may happen to a heavily pregnant woman whose womb presses on the veins in the abdomen.

b. Hypoglycaemic attacks. Although these attacks should seldom be confused with epilepsy, they are relevant. In Chapter 1 (p. 7) very low blood sugar was cited as one of the internal environmental factors which might cause fits in people who did not suffer from epilepsy. Hypoglycaemia may act as a precipitant of seizures in those with epilepsy.

Hypoglycaemia causes symptoms in some patients who have had stomach operations, but these are unlikely to be confused with epilepsy. Attacks which may be so confused occur when there is an excess of insulin (which reduces the level of blood sugar). Most of these are in patients with known diabetes (very rarely with tumours of the glands producing insulin). They may mimic complex partial seizures. At first there are symptoms of disturbance of body functions (autonomic) and later strange behaviour with a state of altered consciousness. There will be a feeling of hunger, sweating, palpitations, a dry mouth and tremor. In a patient known to have diabetes and to be receiving insulin the attack can be stopped almost immediately by giving glucose either by mouth or by injection. When there is an insulin-producing tumour, the diagnosis may be missed

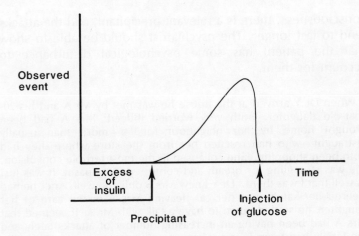

Fig. 3.4 Time scale of a hypoglycaemic attack which builds up slowly, is due to too much insulin, and which can be stopped quickly by an injection of glucose.

and is a matter for specialists. The time scale of a hypo-glycaemic attack is represented in Figure 3.4.

2. Psychological attacks

These are common and account for most of the patients who are misdiagnosed as suffering from epilepsy. Sometimes the diagnosis should be fairly obvious, but often it takes an experienced psychiatrist and perhaps sophisticated EEG tests (p. 79) to determine whether or not an attack is epileptic.

a. Violent outbursts. Sudden catastrophic rages may occur in patients with personality disorders. They should be quite easy to distinguish from epilepsy although confusion may arise if the patient's EEG shows some slight abnormality which is misinterpreted as being due to epilepsy. In these episodes there is some evidence of external provocation, which, although it may be trivial, is relevant. There is no alteration of consciousness and the violence is directed meaningfully.

b. Panic attacks. These may be very difficult to distinguish from complex partial seizures, since in both cases there are autonomic disturbances—sweating, choking feelings, pounding of the heart, etc.—and feelings of fear or acute anxiety. However, in panic attacks there is no true alteration of consciousness, there is a relevant precipitant, and the attacks tend to last longer. The psychiatrist should be able to show that the patient has some psychological disturbance to account for them.

When Dr Y arrived at the house he was met by Mr A and his 20-year-old daughter: both very worried indeed. Mrs A had been brought home by her neighbour Mrs B—more than usually distraught—who had rescued her from the store where they had both been shopping. 'She collapsed in the most terrible convulsion. she was struggling for breath and contorted into spasm. It was just as well that I was there.' Dr Y knew Mrs B only too well. After he had steered her safely into her car, leaving Mrs A in the care of her daughter, he settled down to have a talk with Mr A. It seemed that Mrs A had been having an increasing number of attacks lately and the family had been trying to persuade her to go to see Dr Y. She was all right at home but became more and more tense when she was out and about. Often she became overcome with an intense fear. Several times she had rushed out of a shop without buying anything because she was terrified of passing out.

Later Dr Y questioned Mrs A, who by this time was calm and fully recovered. She confirmed what her husband had said. Yes, she had had several faints. This last time she had a sudden feeling of over-whelming fear, of panic. She felt lightheaded and strange, she felt as if she was outside her own body, she felt that everything around her was distorted in shape and size, she felt as if she was suffocating. She was panting for breath. Her hands and feet were tingling and then they went all stiff. She must have passed out. She could hear people talking all round her. Yes, she remembered quite distinctly hearing Mrs B talk about convulsions and epilepsy.

Mrs A was most distressed by her attacks and was only too happy to accept Dr Y's referral to the psychiatric unit in the nearby teaching hospital. They confirmed what Dr Y had suspected, an acute anxiety state with fears (phobias) particularly of public places. She made a good recovery after a long period of psychological treatment.

Comment

Mrs A was lucky to have a good GP who knew her well and had the time to take a careful history. Her attacks might well have been misdiagnosed as complex partial seizures. There are clues to the correct diagnosis: the feeling of fear or panic, the gradual onset, and her awareness of what was happening even after her collapse. Incidentally she did not have convulsions. In her panic she overbreathed and this caused changes in blood gases which resulted in tingling and tetanic spasms of her extremities. There were two other possible pitfalls. People with epilepsy are quite liable to have anxiety attacks in public places for fear of making an exhibition of themselves in a true seizure (p. 102). Had Mrs A had an EEG done, this might well have shown minor slow wave abnormalities, perhaps over a temporal lobe, and these might have been misinterpreted as epilepsy (p. 79).

c. Feigned fits. This terms is used to cover attacks which although they mimic epileptic fits are not associated with the appropriate electrical disturbance of brain function. They range from the fit deliberately acted out by the malingerer for obvious gain, to the truly hysterical fit produced subconsciously outwith the patient's control. Apart from the malingerer the feigned fit is a cry for help whether at a conscious or unconscious level.

These attacks may present great difficulties in diagnosis, particularly since they occur commonly in patients who have some degree of brain damage, and because patients who suffer from epilepsy are liable to have additional feigned fits, the more so when they are overdosed with antiepileptic drugs. There are some useful distinguishing points. Feigned attacks occur before an audience. The movements tend to be exaggerated and spectacular, representing the patient's idea of what a 'really good fit' should look like. Injury is uncommon, and they are made worse by attempts to restrain the patient, and improve if he is ignored. As with other forms of psychological attack it is important for the psychiatrist to be able to demonstrate positively some underlying mental upset. EEG recordings during an attack are of great value (p. 79).

Miss de V. was 23, she lived in the West country, and she was engaged to be married to a boy from the bank. Everything seemed to be going well for her. When she was 10 months old she had a throat infection with a high fever. She had a prolonged convulsion since it took some time for the doctor to arrive. All went well until she was 11 when she started to have seizures. These always started on the left side but soon they developed to tonic-clonic convulsions. She was treated with phenytoin and her attacks were quite well controlled. Her fiancé and everyone in the village knew about her occasional attacks and neither she nor anyone else worried about them over much. She did quite well at school and when she left she helped out in her father's little grocery shop. She hated the work and sometimes wondered whether she was being over-protected by her parents. She kept feeling that, had she not had fits, she would have been able to have a proper job. Anyway, soon she would be married, she would be free.

However, things started to go a bit wrong. Perhaps it was the excitement, the pressures, the general interest in the forthcoming wedding, and the awareness of the responsibilities she was taking on, the decisions she would need to make. She started to have quite a few more fits. This would never do. She went along to see dear old Dr H, a good friend who had known her since he brought her into the world. He was most understanding. She was having quite a small dose of phenytoin. Why not double it to tide her over the few months before the wedding.

To everyone's consternation the result was disastrous. Her fits got worse rather than better, she became disinterested and unable to make even simple decisions about her future plans. Sensibly Dr H arranged for her referral to neurological out-patients. When she arrived her speech was a bit slurred, she walked rather unsteadily and she seemed to giggle for no apparent reason. She was admitted to hospital.

She appeared to be showing the signs of drug intoxication and blood was taken for estimation of *serum* phenytoin *level*. In the meantime she had a routine EEG examination. During the recording she had several of her attacks. These started with wild movements of the right side of her body but were not accompanied by any change in the EEG record apart from muscle artefact (p. 70). The EEG technician reported this to the house doctor, who did not seem to be very interested. Next day the serum levels were available and showed that Miss de V had a very high phenytoin level, she was severely intoxicated.

This is a tale in which everything ends happily ever after. Her phenytoin was reduced to its previous level, her attacks subsided, she was reassured, and at her wedding those few who had commented: 'Well you know what it is like with epileptics,' were confounded.

Comment

Many points could be made. The one which we want to illustrate is that whereas the first increase in her seizures was due to her natural anxieties, the later attacks were due to intoxication. The EEG technician was correct. They were feigned attacks, quite outwith Miss de V's control. She was not putting them on. She was intoxicated.

3. Other types of attack

a. Special non-epileptic attacks which affect young children will be considered in Chapter 12.

b. Menière's syndrome. The patient, who is usually middle-aged, is seized suddenly with an intense feeling of rotation of his surroundings and he seems to throw himself to the ground. The syndrome is due to a disturbance of the inner ear and can be distinguished from epilepsy because between attacks there will be increasing deafness and buzzing in the ears.

c. Lack of blood to the brain stem. This results in loss of consciousness and occurs either as a rather unusual form of migraine or because the blood vessels supplying the brain stem get pinched as they pass through the bones of the neck. The latter type usually occurs in older people, when they make sudden movements of the head, because other blood vessels which might provide an alternative supply of blood are also narrowed. These attacks can be distinguished because before consciousness is lost there will be disturbances of other functions of the brain stem: for example, double vision, unsteadiness of gait or poor articulation of speech.

Investigation to try to find a cause for the epilepsy.

Having established that the attack was a seizure it is essential for the doctor to make sure that it is not due to a remediable lesion. It is very important to appreciate, and so be able to explain to the patient, that there is no uniform system of investigation of fits. The extent of the investigations will depend on the individual patient, the results of early examination and the doctor's estimate of the probability that a test will show a useful positive reslt. However, because one tonic-clonic convulsion is like another, it is difficult, let us say, for a mother to understand this. Her Johnny, aged two, 'was not treated right,' not like Mrs Sinclair's Susan, aged two months who had 'proper doctors in the hospital.' Johnny, who had always been healthy, had a tummy upset with a high temperature and had a brief febrile convulsion. Susan was clearly a very ill baby. She was admitted to hospital where it was thought at first that she had some biochemical disorder of the blood which had provoked her seizure. When the blood tests were normal a specimen of brain fluid (cerebrospinal fluid, csf) was obtained by *lumbar puncture.** The csf showed that she had meningitis. We will consider in very general terms the various stages of the investigations.

---

* Lumbar punctures are only exceptionally necessary when seizures are being investigated. Susan was one of the exceptions. Meningitis is difficult to diagnose in infants.

1. The General Practitioner

Provided that he can get a good history from someone who has seen the attack, the GP will usually be able to eliminate those which were not epileptic. Unless the patient lives a long way away from hospital, or the GP has a special interest in epilepsy, it is sensible that patients should be referred to hospital to confirm the diagnosis and carry out routine tests. A possible exception would be a short febrile convulsion in a previously healthy child.

2. Simple routine investigation

a. History from a competent observer. In most cases the confirmation of the diagnosis will depend on the history. Further detailed description may suggest that a tonic-clonic seizure started as a simple partial motor attack and this would alert the doctor to the possibility of a brain lesion.

b. Physical examination. In most cases this will show nothing but sometimes it will provide important clues. For example:

Physical sign	A clue to
local weakness	a brain lesion
one side of the body smaller than the other	damage to the opposite side of the brain at an early age
a 'port-wine' stain on the face	Sturge-Weber syndrome (p. 16).

c. Blood tests. Although routine examination of blood constituents is unlikely to show positive results except in infants, in most hospitals it is automated and should be done for the records.

d. Skull x-ray. Only rarely will there be a positive result but then it will be of great importance as suggesting the presence of a tumour.

e. Chest x-ray. Lung tumours are very common and often spread to the brain. Therefore, this should be a routine test in older patients.

f. EEG Although the limitations will be dealt with at the end of this chapter, a baseline record should be done whenever there is an EEG machine available.

3. Further tests which may be necessary

Until fairly recently the tests available to exclude such remediable lesions as tumours or blood clots, involved taking x-rays of the brain after the injection of air (*air encephalogram*) or a dye into one of the arteries supplying the brain (*arteriogram*). Both tests were painful and distressing for the patient, they required his admission to hospital for several days and they carried an appreciable risk. Neurologists therefore had to use all their skill and experience to weigh up whether the possibility of finding a remediable lesion warranted subjecting the patient to discomfort, inconvenience and even danger.

Nowadays, air encephalograms and arteriograms are only carried out as part of highly specialized investigations prior to surgery for the relief of epilepsy (p. 64). They have been replaced by brain scans and, in particular, *computerized tomography* (*CT scan*). This test involves the taking of large numbers of x-rays at different planes of the brain, feeding these pictures to a computer and obtaining very accurate maps of the brain. Even more sophisticated variations are being developed. The CT scan is painless, without danger and can be done in an out-patient department. It is, however, expensive and it is not available in all hospitals.

The CT scan has revolutionized the further investigation of epilepsy and there is now a tendency in some units to use it rather too much; 'just to be on the safe side', or even for general interest to find out what is causing seizures, although there is no real likelihood of showing a lesion which requires treatment. This wider use of the CT scan has been useful in increasing doctors' understanding of epilepsy and, in particular, has reduced further the number of seizures previously considered to be primary—not due to brain damage. However, it is important that the patient should understand this change in emphasis. He needs to be reassured that, if he is called for further special investigations, this does not mean necessarily that the specialist suspects some sinister and dangerous condition, or that he may be subject later to operation.

It is worth considering some of the clues which in the past would have made an air encephalogram or an arteriogram necessary, and which now would make the alternative CT scan mandatory.

   a. Age. Blood clots can result from head injuries at any age. Otherwise they occur with vascular accidents (p. 16). These are usually obvious, although clots form on the surface of the brain in old patients after comparatively minor injuries. These can be missed if a CT scan is not done.

Brain tumours very rarely cause seizures in children or adolescents: in adults there are usually some other clues (see below).

   b. Type of seizure. Simple absences, which can be diagnosed definitively by the EEG are a form of primary epilepsy and do not need further investigation.

Complex partial seizures are due occasionally to tumours but are much more likely to be the result of a difficult birth or prolonged febrile convulsions. If there is a history of either and there are no other clues, special tests are less necessary.

Simple partial seizures are much more likely to be due to a remediable lesion, unless there is a clear history of a localized head injury—such as a wartime gunshot wound.

   c. Evidence from earlier examinations of localized brain dysfunction.

 (i) The history suggested that a seizure started in one part of the body

 (ii) Physical examination showed evidence of local weakness or loss of sensation.

 (iii) The skull x-ray was abnormal.

 (iv) The EEG gave a clue that between seizures there was a localized abnormality.

 (v) If the chest x-ray has shown lung cancer, there would be a strong presumption that the seizures were due to spread to the brain. Since there is no effective treatment at this stage, the patient should not be subjected to the anxiety and false hopes of further investigations.

Is the drug treatment suitable?

Epilepsy has been confirmed. A remediable cause for the recurrent seizures has been excluded. The patient now needs the best possible medical treatment in order to control his fits. It is important for him to appreciate that some are controlled more easily than others and that if they continue it is not necessarily his doctor's fault. If he does not understand, there is a real danger that he will press for more and more anti-epileptic drugs to control his fits 'at any cost.' All too often the cost is too high (Ch. 8). Other patients or their families, frustrated by continuing seizures, will go from one doctor to another seeking a solution to an insoluble problem.

With the best possible treatment many patients with epilepsy can have their seizures controlled either completely or with only occasional attacks. Others cannot. Two general points must be made:

1. As explained in Chapter 1, the greater the element of brain sensitivity and the less that of brain damage, the more effective are antiepileptic drugs. The uncommon simple absences can usually be controlled quite well although they may not be stopped altogether; as can the rare primary generalized tonic-clonic convulsions

2. Complex partial seizures are notoriously difficult to treat, although they may be controlled partially with one of the more recent drugs (carbamazepine). However, it is usually possible to prevent such seizures developing to major fits (p. 66). Complex partial seizures, although inconvenient and often an important social disability, are not dangerous, and it may be better to settle for preventing their development to major fits, and then to ignore them. This policy is in itself often effective, since such seizures are probably precipitated by the anxiety that they may happen. Furthermore, they are particularly likely to be increased rather than reduced by over-enthusiastic efforts to control them with large doses of drugs.

There remains the important situation when the patient and his non-medical adviser have very good reason to believe that the treatment is not suitable. Both feel that something needs to be done but are wary of antagonizing the doctor involved— of being classified as 'difficult.' Each situation needs to be dealt with individually, but often it is possible tactfully to suggest that: 'Mr. X is a bit worried about his seizures, do you think it would reassure him and relieve the pressure on you if you referred him back to the hospital consultant?' Put in the right way, the doctor himself often will be only too relieved to do so.

The place of surgical treatment

Even after suitable medical treatment has been organized there will remain quite a large percentage of patients who still have fits. Chronic seizures represent an important disadvantage, and to some a serious social and psychological disability. It is not surprising that patients, frustrated and desperate, should seek any way of stopping their fits. Some will have heard or read of successful surgical treatment: a form of treatment which has an especial appeal since it cuts out, extirpates, that evil part which is poisoning their lives.

There is no doubt that in certain patients surgery can stop or alleviate seizures. However, this group is small (Fig. 3.1), and it is important to appreciate the limitations of surgery in order to be able to advise patients: to avoid the additional frustration and dejection of hopes unfulfilled.

We have emphasized the two factors which together result in recurrent seizures: brain sensitivity and brain damage. In very general and much over-simplified terms, antiepileptic drugs can help to reduce brain sensitivity, whereas surgical excision may possibly be able to remove a piece of damaged brain. Before surgery should be considered, certain criteria need to be satisfied. Some are medically technical. General criteria can be appreciated more easily.

1. It must have proved impossible to control seizures adequately with antiepileptic drugs.

a. Although no miracle drugs have been discovered recently, a great deal has been found out over the past few years about the correct way of using existing drugs (Ch. 8). Not all doctors are aware of these developments. The patient must be assessed in a specialized unit.

b. For one reason or another many patients do not take the drugs which have been prescribed for them (patient *compliance*). It may even be necessary to admit a patient to hospital or to a Special Centre for Epilepsy to check on his compliance.

c. Seizures are sensitive not only to the internal environment of drug levels, but also to the external environment of psychological and social pressures (Ch. 7). It is often helpful for a patient to spend some time in a special unit to assess what control may be achieved by adequate control of this external environment.

2. It is important to make sure that a patient's remaining seizures do represent a sufficient disability to warrant subjecting him to an operation which carries a small but significant further risk of disability or even death. The decision will depend on the degree to which these seizures interrupt his life and work. An accountant with frequent complex partial seizures might be contrasted with a gardener whose occasional seizures were accepted by his employer.

3. It needs to be determined whether a patient with additional handicaps would benefit from a major operation which, attempting to eliminate his fits, would have no material effect on his other problems. It is usually felt that those with a significant degree of mental handicap—say an IQ of under 70—are not suitable for operation.

Further criteria depend on the neurosurgeon being able to demonstrate that there is brain damage which can be removed without causing important loss of brain function: and further, that the brain damage is localized and that there are not other parts of the brain which may later give rise to seizures.

Operations for the relief of epilepsy can be divided into three groups:

1. The removal of small areas of the surface of the brain (cerebral cortex) which are causing simple partial seizures. In most cases such operations will have been carried out because of lesions requiring treatment in their own right (p. 59). Rarely, there may be local lesions produced, say, from head or gunshot wounds, which although not in themselves dangerous, can be removed for the relief of fits.

2. Complex operations are being developed experimentally to destroy deep parts of the brain considered to be involved in seizures. We need not consider such operations further.

3. The removal of part of the temporal lobe for the relief of complex partial seizures. These account for the great majority of surgical interventions. In expert hands they are often successful and we will consider them briefly.

a. The patients who do best are those who have a history of a particular type of damage to the deep parts of the temporal lobe from either prolonged febrile convulsions, or, less commonly birth injury.

b. Special investigations must be carried out to make sure that there is not similar damage to the other temporal lobe.

If there is, the removal of one lobe may cause serious permanent memory problems.

c. Patients with behavioural and personality disturbances, clearly secondary to their epilepsy, do well when seizures are controlled by operation. Those with primary psychiatric disorders or mental handicap are not helped and should not be operated on.

d. These operations should be carried out only in units specialized not only in surgical techniques, but more importantly in the choice of patients suitable for operation.

The prognosis is not one of doom

The different stages which have been worked through in this chapter should make it possible for someone helping or advising the patient with epilepsy to reassure him that faced with the diagnosis, epilepsy, is not to present a diagnosis of doom. Nevertheless, there remains a significant group of patients who continue to have fits. To advise them sensibly it is necessary to have some idea of prognosis so that reassurance does not lose credibility through over-enthusiasm.

1. Many statistics relate to times when the correct use of antiepileptic drugs was not understood fully. There are still all too many patients with continuing seizures, which could be controlled better if they had more up-to-date and experienced advice.

2. As explained in Chapter 1. the population of patients with epilepsy is heterogeneous, and fits are caused in varying degree by brain sensitivity and brain damage. Brain sensitivity is more easily treated with drugs, brain damage is amenable occasionally to surgery.

a. The prognosis for the severely brain damaged patient with significant mental handicap is not good.

b. That for the child with brain sensitive simple absences is very good.

c. It is difficult to control complex partial seizures, due to brain damage, unless they are in the small group suitable for temporal lobectomy. However, the tendency for complex partial seizures to develop to secondary generalized tonic-clonic convulsions is very probably due to the factor of brain sensitivity, and this development is easier to control.

3. Increasingly it is appreciated that fits uncontrolled will cause secondary disturbances of brain function which will make further fits more probable. It is most undesirable to treat 'attacks' which may not be epilepsy with antiepileptic drugs. However, once the diagnosis of epilepsy has been made definitively, prompt and adequate treatment will prevent the liability to epilepsy becoming established. If in the future all those with epilepsy are treated in the best possible way, the unfortunate group of those with perisistent seizures should be reduced even further: the prognosis should not be one of doom.

The EEG

A seizure is caused by the uncontrolled activity of groups of brain cells, which results in excessive fluctuations in electrical voltage. The excesses are, however, Lilliputian: measured in millionths of a volt (*microvolts*). The EEG machine, however complex or expensive it may be, is simply an amplifier which magnifies these fluctuations some million times, so that, converted to volts, they can power ink-writing pens to move up and down, and are recorded on moving paper in the form of waves. The height of the wave measures the change in voltage, its width the time during which this change occurs.

In the great majority of cases the EEG can record on paper the explosion which is the seizure. There can be no doubt but that the discovery of the EEG represented one of the most important advances in the understanding of epilepsy. For the first time the inexplicable seizure could be seen to be something which actually happened: a disorder of the brain, not an aberration of the mind, not an event beyond ordinary understanding. Unfortunately, initial enthusiasms led to claims which gave the EEG a bad reputation among doctors, who, not understanding what it was all about, were only too ready to comment on its limitations while failing to appreciate its usefulness.

A routine EEG examination is simple, painless and without risk. It takes about an hour and can be carried out as an outpatient. The apparatus may appear formidable and frightening, but, except for the very young, the very old or the confused patient, any anxieties can be allayed without difficulty by the referring doctor or the EEG technician. Electrical contact is made with 21 pads (*electrodes*) held in standard positions on the scalp by a cap made of thin rubber tubes. The voltage fluctuations between pairs of electrodes are recorded as lines (*channels*) of waves on the moving paper. Various combinations of electrodes ensure that a record covers a wide area of the brain's surface. Towards the end of the test the patient is asked to breathe deeply for three minutes, since the resulting changes in the blood gases (p. 33) often provoke abnormalities not seen in the main record. Other special methods of provocation may be used. It takes some time to place the electrodes and set up the machine. The actual recording time is rather over half an hour. Since the paper usually runs at 3 cm per second the completed record runs to some 40 metres. With a minimum of 8 channels to the page the doctor responsible for interpreting the EEG has to digest about a quarter of a kilometre of information. There are many sophisticated methods of analysing all this information, but for ordinary clinical work most EEG laboratories rely on the personal experience of the reporter. For routine clinical, as against research, work this is sensible. Expert scientific electro-neuro-physiologists have suggested explanations for the production of the EEG's 'brain waves:' Presently, practical interpretation is essentially empirical: based on experience rather than theory.

The normal record

If EEGs are recorded from large numbers of healthy adults the great majority show wave forms which vary within quite narrow limits: these are considered to represent the normal record. When the subject is relaxed with his eyes shut, the main waves or rhythms are recorded from the back of the head. Voltage changes of around 50 microvolts occur about 10 times a second. If he opens his eyes these waves (the *alpha rhythm*) will disappear or be reduced considerably. A typical normal record is shown in Figure 3.5, and one channel of alpha rhythm is reproduced for comparison at the bottom of the other EEG examples. Other normal rhythms are of no particular importance to the understanding of this chapter.

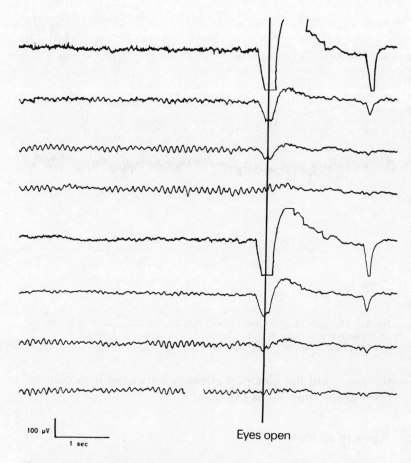

100 µV
1 sec

Eyes open

Fig. 3.5 A normal record showing the reduction of rhythms on opening eyes. For this and other figures in this chapter see also legend for 1.1.

Artefacts

The amplification necessary to record the minute brain waves is so great that it is liable to amplify and record even slight electrical events which occur outside the brain. These unwanted and often confusing parts of the record are called artefacts. It often requires a good deal of experience to distinguish them. Some of the more obvious and important are shown in Figure 3.6: movement of the head, movements of

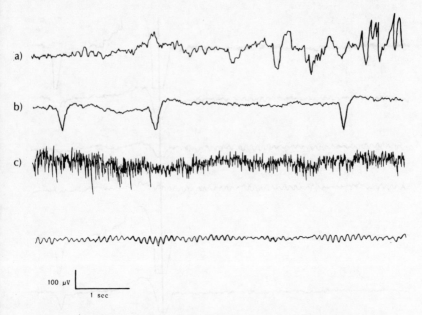

a)

b)

c)

100 μV

1 sec

Fig. 3.6 Artefacts. (a) Movement which may be difficult to distinguish from an abnormality coming from the brain. (b) Eye blinks. (c) Deflections produced by contraction of scalp muscles.

the eyes, and the electrical changes associated with contractions of the muscles of the scalp.

Types of abnormality

1. Spikes and sharp waves. These are voltage changes, often relatively large, which happen very quickly—the spikes more quickly than the sharp waves. Since they are 'sudden excessive fluctuations' (p. 67) they are very suggestive of epilepsy (Fig. 3.7).

2. Localized slow wave abnormalities. These are waves which are of higher voltage and longer duration than the alpha rhythm. They are less regular and they do not form a repetitive rhythm. The severity of this type of abnormality is determined by the size of the waves, how often they occur and how widely they extend over the head. Figure 3.8. shows a mild abnormality, Figure 3.9. a severe one.

3. Generalized abnormalities. These are widespread over

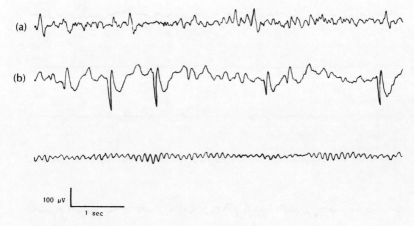

Fig. 3.7 (a) Sharp waves. (b) Spikes: note similarity to 3.6.(a).

the brain and are seen in all or most of the EEG channels. The waves are slower and usually larger than the alpha rhythm, they are regular and rhythmic and they tend to be much less affected by opening the eyes. They suggest an important disorder of the internal environment (p. 4) and are of particular importance in epilepsy as providing a clue that a patient may be having too large a dose of antiepileptic drugs (be intoxicated) (Fig. 3.11).

4. Paroxysmal abnormalities. There is a sudden change in the record which lasts several seconds. Most often the change is one of greatly increased voltage, often with large slow waves and associated spikes (Fig. 1.1). They are very suggestive of epilepsy.

Basic principles

1. The EEG brain waves are produced by masses of living nerve cells: the normal record from normal cells; the abnormal from those which are not functioning properly. Dead parts of the brain—as, for example, after an old injury—are not capable of causing electrical changes.

2. It follows that the EEG measures function (or dysfunction) and not changes in brain structure. When methods of further investigation were limited to the potentially dangerous arteriograms and air encephalograms, the harmless EEG was

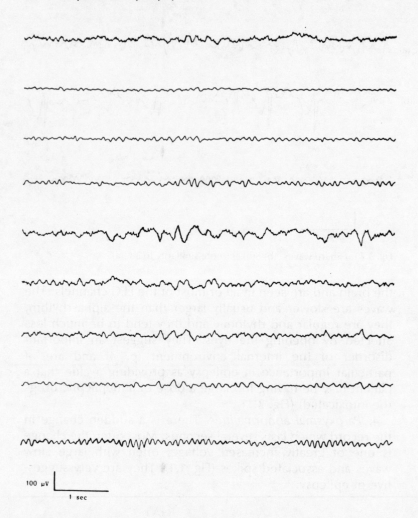

100 μV

1 sec

Fig. 3.8 A mild slow wave abnormality localized to the left side.

used in an attempt to demonstrate structural lesions. Its failure was to be expected, but such improper use did much to impair it's credibility.

3. In the great majority of cases all that the EEG can hope to do is to show that something is wrong in a part or the whole of the brain. It very seldom is able to make the diagnosis. It should not be expected to do so.

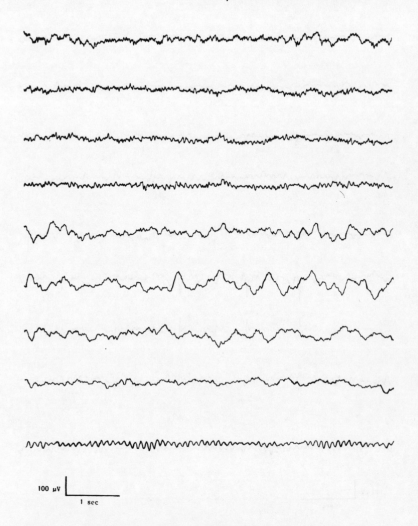

Fig. 3.9 A severe slow wave abnormality localized to the left side.

Some examples of the value of the EEG

1. Simple absences—the EEG during an absence is character-istic (Fig. 2.8). Arising from a normal record, there is a sudden paroxysm of generalized regular high voltage slow waves, each accompanied by a spike at the rate of about three per second. The absence usually lasts from about 10 seconds and

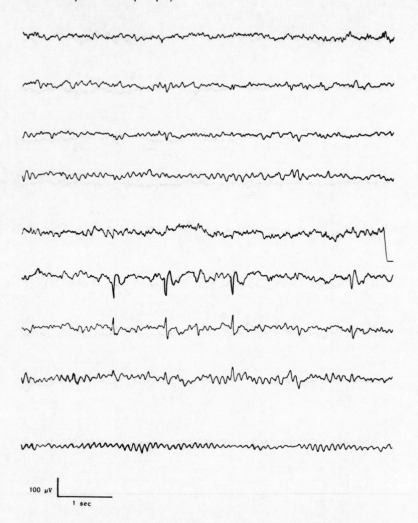

Fig. 3.10 The right side is normal. On the left side there are spike discharges from the temporal lobe suggesting that the patient has complex partial seizures.

the EEG technician should be able to notice some change in the child—perhaps a look of vagueness, possibly some flickering of the eyelids. The EEG is recording a simple absence which might have been missed and it defines the diagnosis.

Children with a clear history of probable absences will often have much briefer paroxysms with no noticeable changes at the time of the paroxysm. If the history is clear and there are such paroxysms, it is highly likely that the child does suffer from absences. The paroxysms are particularly liable to be provoked by the changes in the blood gases resulting from deep breathing.

Since children who do suffer from simple absences are very likely to have longer or shorter paroxysms in their EEGs, if there are no paroxysms in the EEG, it would be rather unlikely that the child does have absences.

However, there is a caveat. Relatives of people with epilepsy, and possibly others, may show paroxysms in their EEGs without suffering from simple absences. The findings of paroxysms in a routine EEG does not make for the diagnosis unless either there is a history strongly suggesting absences or the changes associated with absences are noticed at the time of the paroxysms. It is worth emphasizing that simple absences are not as common as it used to be thought.

2. If a patient has a history of attacks of loss of consciousness suggestive of epilepsy, and an EEG showing spikes (Fig. 3.7.) or a paroxysm (Fig. 1.1.), the EEG would support strongly the diagnosis of epilepsy.

3. Complex absences —it may be difficult to distinguish absences which occur as a manifestation of very slight complex partial seizures from simple absences (p. 42). If absences have been observed and the EEG shows a pattern as in Figure 3.10, which is suggestive of a complex partial seizure arising from the left temporal lobe, it is evident that the patient suffers from complex partial seizures rather than simple absences. The distinction is important since the treatment and the prognosis are different.

4. If between seizures the EEG shows evidence of a localized slow wave abnormality (Fig. 3.9), this would suggest local brain damage which might need to be investigated further (p. 62).

5. Although generalized EEG changes (Fig. 3.11) are nonspecific in that they are not diagnostic of any particular condition, they do indicate a disturbance of the internal environment. For patients with epilepsy they often give a clue to intoxication with an excessive dose of drugs.

6. Unusual types of status (or serial) epilepticus have been mentioned. The EEG will be crucial in these cases in distin-

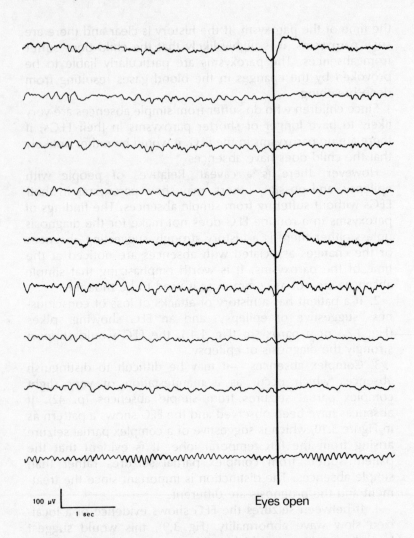

100 µV

1 sec

Eyes open

Fig. 3.11 A generalized abnormality. The waves are rather larger and slower than normal and they are little affected by opening the eyes.

guishing whether the observed alteration of behaviour is due to epileptic activity as against a psychiatric disturbance.

7. Special EEG tests can be helpful when brain surgery is being considered. If a part of the brain is to be removed to control fits, it is necessary to show not only that there are abnormal discharges from the part to be removed, but also

that no such discharges are present in the brain that is left. This applies particularly to removal of a part of one temporal lobe. If the other lobe is damaged, the patient would be left without effective temporal lobes, with consequent serious memory disorders.

8. Many patients with severe epilepsy, who are in hospitals or institutions, have very severe EEG abnormalities which can be contrasted easily with a normal record. These same patients may have serious behaviour disorders which try the patience of the nurses and auxilliaries who are looking after them. If they can see the objective evidence of the EEG, it is often easier for them to consider their charges, not as wilful or bloody-minded, but rather as patients in need of help.

Some examples of the limitations of the EEG

1. If only a small volume of brain is involved in a partial seizure (simple or complex) or if the part is remote from the electrodes which record from the surface of the brain, there may be no EEG changes even during a seizure. However, this is exceptional and in the great majority of patients the EEG will show characteristic changes during and immediately after a fit.

2. However, epilepsy is an episodic condition and some patients have seizures only very occasionally. The limitations of the EEG are mainly when records are carried out between seizures. The routine recording lasts only about half an hour and the chances of a fit during this time are very slight, particularly since the patient is likely to be a bit tense and anxious—a state which often suppresses fits. We will consider the value of a single routine record.

a. The record is normal. This does not in any way exclude epilepsy.

b. Paroxysms are found sometimes in routine records when there is no history suggestive of epilepsy. In this event the EEG is not enough to make the diagnosis of epilepsy—at most it might mean that the patient has a higher than average degree of brain sensitivity and is rather more likely to develop epilepsy should he suffer brain damage.

c. Patients with a history of the psychological attacks described on page 55 often have EEGs carried out as a routine and it is quite common to find minor slow wave irregularities.

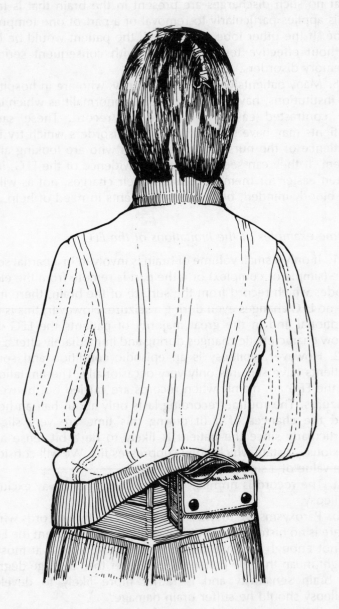

Fig. 3.12 A girl fitted with Medilog equipment showing the electrodes on her head and the recording box attached to a belt round her waist.

These must not be misinterpreted as suggesting that the attacks are epileptic.

d. Spike or paroxysmal discharges recorded between attacks provide only a very rough guide to the severity of a patient's epilepsy—the frequency of his attacks. It often happens, particularly with complex partial seizures, that the EEG is quite abnormal when the seizures are well controlled, and much less abnormal when attacks are frequent.

Ambulatory recording (Medilog)

The main value of the EEG is to record what happens during an attack. If there are no EEG changes during an attack, which is other than very slight (see above), this is very strong evidence that the attack is not epileptic. One of the most important recent advances in EEG work has been the system whereby the EEG can be recorded, if necessary for days, until an attack occurs. Small electrodes are fixed firmly to the patient's head and lead discreetly to a tape recorder which he carries on a strap round his waist (Fig. 3.12). He is able to carry on with all his normal activities. There is a special button which can be pressed when an attack occurs and this makes a signal on the tape. Although there are some technical difficulties, the method is likely to prove of great value.

There is one important caution. As with all forms of EEG work the *Medilog* does not provide an automatic diagnosis. As we explained on page 57, patients who suffer from epilepsy are particularly likely to have feigned or hysterical attacks in addition to their epileptic seizures. If the Medilog is normal during an attack, all that can be said with certainty is that that particular attack was not an epileptic one. It is not possible to say that the patient does not suffer from epilepsy. However, the more often feigned attacks can be recorded, and the more they resemble other attacks which he has, the less likely it is that he does suffer from epilepsy.

4

What should I do when he has a fit?

This is almost always the first question that relatives, friends and associates ask. It is essential, therefore, that those who are to advise and help, should be able to give a clear and authoritative answer. This chapter is concerned with the circumstances of the fit itself. More general problems of coping with epilepsy will be considered later (Ch. 7). However, it is not enough to be able to explain all about seizures and to hand out a pamphlet of *Do's* and *Don't's*. It is necessary first to understand and sympathize with the effect of the seizure on the observer. The closer his relationship to the patient the more devastating the impact will be. There is often a state of shock which negates reassurance and confuses instructions. To tell the mother, wife or husband, desperately worried and often terrified, that there is nothing to worry about, that there is nothing special which needs to be done, is as useless as to try to stop a seizure by the laying on of hands.

Doctors, and particularly neurologists who deal with many patients with epilepsy, may be too well-informed, too aware that epilepsy is not a disaster, to go along with the apparently irrational attitude of the patient's family. It is here that the paramedical adviser has such an important role to play. If she can understand the initial impact, the shock, she can help the family to work through their early reaction to the point when her reassurance will be acceptable and her practical instructions understood.

Before advising on the immediate management of different types of seizures it is worth considering three quite different aspects of attacks which cause great distress to the family observer: the horror of the tonic-clonic convulsion, the inexplicability of the complex partial seizure, and the inevitability, particularly, of the major fit.

1. The horror

To witness a tonic-clonic convulsion for the first time, or even for the second or third time, is an awesome and terrible experience. The person, known so well, is contorted and distorted, becomes almost like a wild animal or a rabid dog. Soon he passes into a coma from which he cannot be roused. To the lay person he seems to be dead. The doctor knows that this phase will pass in 5 or 10 minutes. The mother 'knows' that her child is dead.

2. The inexplicability

Often the drama and horror of the major fit may be easier to accept and understand than the more subtle and inexplicable behaviour seen in some complex partial seizures.

To wake one morning to find that half of the roof has been blown down in a storm is a catastrophe: but it can be seen as such. To wake to find that there is an aspidistra where the tea-making machine used to be, and that there are tadpoles in the glass of water by your bed, can be far more terrifying: it is not reasonable: are you, perhaps, going mad?

'William, my solid sensible husband, seems to be behaving quite inappropriately. In the sitting room with some friends, he was talking normally: or was he? Perhaps we have all had too many drinks. But, no: he is talking to someone in the corner, who is not there. What he is saying does not seem to make much sense. I did not hear properly. I was trying to make out what George was saying. What was that? William has just belched and I am sure I heard him fart—but he seems quite unconcerned. He does look a little strange. He is pale and sweating, but then the room is a bit hot. Yes, he is hot. He is taking off his coat and fumbling with the zip of his trousers. Am I mad? Is he mad? Where is the aspidistra? Who are the tadpoles? No, it is all right. He has settled down and is quiet, he seems to be talking quietly to himself—no just mumbling. Perhaps, it was just me. I wonder. He seems embarrassed and is trying to do up his zip without anyone noticing. He takes little part in the rest of the evening's conversation but he is able to say good-bye to our friends. What did they think? What do I think? He did not know!'

3. The inevitability

We know, and you know, that almost every seizure is self-limiting and is only most exceptionally dangerous. The family observer finds this very difficult to accept, even after many experiences. As we have written before (Laidlaw and Laidlaw, 1982), to watch a tonic-clonic convulsion is nightmarish. 'You have just got the baby to sleep when a strident alarm clock goes off. It is out of reach. If you could think clearly, you would know that it would stop in two minutes, but it seems to blare away for an eternity, and there is nothing that you can do to stop it!' It is so important that the observer should have the reassurance of knowing exactly what he should and what he should not do. It is even worth over-emphasizing the *do's*: the observer needs help as much as the patient.

Different types of fits present different requirements for immediate management. However, in every case it is important that the observer should record and report to the doctor a careful description. This will sometimes help the doctor to make his diagnosis. More often, after several seizures the diagnosis will have been made already, but the sensible doctor will accept these reports graciously, not dismissing them as evidence of neurotic and obsessional relatives, but rather appreciating that he is treating, not fits, but the much larger problem of the Family Seizure.

Simple absences

There are brief self-limiting attacks, without danger of injury, and which do not develop into the potentially dangerous tonic-clonic convulsion. There is, therefore, nothing which needs to be done during the brief absence.

Absences may be very frequent and may interfere seriously with a child's life. Parents or teachers must understand that in such cases failure to do what he is told does not mean that the child is wilful or disobedient but often that he was just 'not there'—absent. In school the child with repeated absences will be classified, all too easily, as stupid. In fact the range of intelligence for these children is just the same as for any other child. It is most frustrating for a bright child wrongly to be treated as unintelligent and such treatment is more than likely to increase the number of absences and to make matters even worse.

Simple partial seizures

It is rather unusual for these attacks to remain localized. Most of them develop to secondary tonic-clonic convulsions. If they do not spread, no immediate action is necessary, but the patient must be referred to a doctor, since there may be a causative lesion which needs treatment. For the same reason if they do spread, it is important for the observer to note and report the beginning of the seizure so that the doctor is aware that the convulsion is not a primary one.

Complex partial seizures

Often these attacks will develop quickly into tonic-clonic convulsions. The patient may be aware of the early part of the attack as his warning (aura) or the observer may come to recognize alterations in appearance or behaviour which presage the big attack. As with simple partial seizures these early signs should be passed on to the doctor.

Once treatment with antiepileptic drugs has been started many attacks will not develop and the observer will need a great deal of understanding to deal with them. The patient is not unconscious but rather in a state of altered consciousness. He is not responsible for his actions and it is impossible to reason with him as with a rational and fully conscious person. On the other hand, he retains some degree of awareness and an albeit impaired and distorted ability to react to his environment. Two consequences of this penumbria of consciousness are illustrative.

1. A patient should never be restrained during a seizure—of whatever type—unless he is at risk of injury. This applies particularly in this type of attack. His semi-automatic, semi-purposive behaviour may be not only inappropriate but a practical embarrassment. 'He is putting my knitting into the washing up bowl.' To attempt to restrain him would be disastrous. He is not able to understand restraint or interference. Complex partial seizures involve parts of the brain concerned with emotions, particularly those of fear. Any interference would be liable to evoke terror reactions of violence, as purposeless and undirected as his original behaviour. Patients with epilepsy have a wholly undeserved reputation for violence during their seizures. In almost every case this is based solely on the response of a partially conscious patient to interference of which he is only dimly aware. His reactions to restraint are no more purposeful than are the actions which someone is trying to restrain. They are not directed, they are not dangerous, and they can be avoided so easily by a proper understanding of his experience during a complex partial seizure.

2. A patient subject to complex partial seizures soon realizes that there are occasions when for minutes at a time he loses that ordinary control which he exercises over his environment—periods when, not only is his behaviour not his own behaviour, but periods lost to his consciousness during which he does not know what he has done. Those round him must do everything possible to support and reassure him as he recovers, and, when he is recovered fully, ensure that he finds himself in an atmosphere of calm. Later, he may be helped a great deal more if he is told what did happen during his attack, than if he is surrounded by an ambience of mystery and silence. It would be unusual for his behaviour to have been anything like as unacceptable as he may have feared. The matter of fact acceptance by his friends is the most helpful way in which they can react to this type of seizure.

Tonic-clonic convulsions

Whether these are primary or secondary there is not much that the observer can do to help but there are some essential *do's* and *don't's*. It is important to remember that the patient is completely unconscious; he cannot feel anything and he is quite unable to make any appropriate response.

Do:

1. Prevent him from injuring his head, if without restraint you can put something soft between it and the ground. If there is nothing else available, your foot will be a help.
2. If you can, remove his spectacles and/or false teeth.
3. Ensure that he can breathe as easily as possible.
   a. Loosen anything constricting round his neck.
   b. Turn him over on his side into a position as if he were hugging the floor. Make sure that his head is also turned to one side. It should be lower than the rest of his body. If the tongue seems to be falling back, try to pull it forward and press the jaw upwards. If there is a lot of froth and spit in his mouth, clear this away with a handkerchief.
4. After the worst of the attack is over:
   a. Before he recovers consciousness try to clear up any evidence of incontinence which would embarrass him.
   b. While he is still unconscious and insensitive clean up any superficial abrasions which do not need medical attention.

Do not:

1. Attempt to restrain him unless it is absolutely necessary for his immediate safety.
2. Attempt to put anything into his mouth to prevent him biting his tongue. If he is to bite his tongue, usually he will have done so during the first tonic phase before you have got to his help. The tradition of putting a spoon between his teeth is wholly ill-founded and likely only to damage his teeth.
3. Give him anything to drink. If he is lucky you will fail. If he is unlucky you will choke him.
4. Call a doctor except under the conditions explained below. As a patient recovers from a major fit, he will be confused, only returning slowly to normal consciousness. As he does so he will be reassured by familiar faces and an attitude of

calm. If the seizure has been at all severe, he will be exhausted and will want to sleep. He should be allowed to do so. It is usually quite easy to distinguish between someone who is confused and sleepy and a patient who is still deeply unconscious—in coma. The latter will make no responses to those round him.

When should the doctor be called?

The family can be helped a great deal by being given a clear answer to this question.

1. The doctor should always be called after the first seizure and this includes a febrile convulsion in a child.
2. Otherwise the doctor should not be called for any seizure other than a tonic-clonic convulsion, and then only for the following reasons.
   a. If the seizure lasts longer than usual. Patient's seizures vary in length but one lasting more than 10 minutes should be suspect.
   b. If one seizure leads into another without recovery of consciousness in between. There is a serious risk that he is going into a status epilepticus (p. 45) and this is a medical emergency. If the GP is not available a 999 call should be made and he should go into hospital.
   c. If during his seizure he has suffered an injury, which clearly needs medical attention. If there is serious bleeding which cannot be stopped by simple pressure, this is a medical emergency and requires hospital admission as in (b).
   d. If after the seizure is over, he appears to be unrousable and deeply unconscious rather than sleeping. This applies particularly if there is any suggestion that he may have injured his head during the seizure.

There is one other contingency which needs to be considered. A few patients, even with the best possible treatment remain subject to repeated tonic-clonic convulsions. The seizures themselves may be relatively mild and self-limiting but should they occur among those who do not understand them, they are liable to cause consternation and result in the ambulance being called and the patient being sent unnecessarily to hospital. It would be no restriction on such a person's liberty, if he was advised not to venture out in public unaccompanied by someone who understood his liability to seizures. If this is not practicable, he should be advised to carry some identification, such as Medicalert (p. 74) which would save everyone a great deal of disruption.

REFERENCE

Laidlaw M V, Laidlaw J 1982 Epilepsy explained. Churchill Livingstone, Edinburgh

5

The exorcism of the epileptic personality

'Pedantic, egocentric, religiose, suspicious, adhesive, quarrel-some, aggressive, and so on and so forth'.

These pejorative adjectives were not attributed to 'The epileptic' in bygone days when The Devil was suspected strongly of having a hand in the causation of seizures. As recently as a generation ago they were presented in respected psychiatric texts as defining the epileptic personality, the inevitable consequence of having seizures. At just about the same time as penicillin was revolutionizing the treatment of infections, this latter day devilish concept was one of the most important foundations of both medical and popular prejudice against epilepsy. Sadly, the concept, like any prejudice, is slow in dying and still lingers on in the more obscure mental hospitals, where the nursing staff see in their long-stay patients what they expect to see, and report to their psychiatrists, who do not see these patients very often anyway.

In the next chapter we will consider the general psychological and psychiatric problems of epilepsy. Here we will attempt a final exorcism of the myth of the epileptic personality. To do so, it is important to examine the concept critically. Emotional, albeit well-meaning, propaganda suggesting that all people with epilepsy are angels with immaculate personalities, is so unrealistic it is likely only to perpetuate the myth. Those of us who have to try to help these patients appreciate only too well that there are those who do have problems. We will offer three propositions.

A. There is no personality peculiar to people with epilepsy.

B. Not all people with epilepsy have personality problems.

C. Some people with epilepsy do have personality problems.

If we are to help them we must understand how these have arisen, so that we can help to overcome and avoid them.

It is interesting to follow the changing attitudes to the patient with epilepsy over comparatively recent times.

1. During the mid-19th century epilepsy was classified as a form of insanity. A patient requiring hospital care inevitably received this in an asylum. In England there is a somewhat bizarre legal hang-over. If someone commits a criminal offence for which he was not responsible since it occurred in relation to a seizure, he is considered as not guilty, but insane because he suffers from epilepsy. A respected solicitor while interviewing his client—a comely matron—had one of his rare complex seizures during which he took off his trousers. In theory, because of his indecent exposure, during an epileptic seizure, he might find himself confined indefinitely in Broadmoor—a hospital for the criminally insane. Fortunately 'The Law is not an Ass' and this is unlikely to happen. The patient with epilepsy should be careful nevertheless about adducing epilepsy in his defence. Patients on the Continent or in Scotland have less to fear since they are protected by the wisdom of the Examining Magistrate or the Procurator Fiscal.

2. Some hundred years ago the approach to epilepsy was revolutionized by the emergence of the now world famous National Hospital for Nervous Diseases. Nonetheless, their most eminent neurologists considered that epilepsy led inevitably to a progressive deterioration in intellect and personality. At that time many of their patients may have suffered from brain tumours, and others from the effects of bromide, the only known antiepileptic drug.

3. At the turn of the century descriptive psychiatry was the vogue. Psychiatric illnesses were classified and considered to have a constitutional or hereditary basis. Epilepsy was one

such. It was manifest by characteristic personality changes and by seizures. Those identified as having the appropriate personality profile, even if they did not have fits, were said to be liable to develop them. The Epileptic Personality was born.

4. Later during this century major advances in understanding were made, particularly in the United States. It was appreciated that epilepsy was not a disease in its own right, but rather that seizures were often merely a symptom of some underlying brain damage or disease. Many patients were found to present no personality problems. Some few did have behavioural, intellectual, or personality difficulties, but it was suggested that they might well be due to the effects of a variety of adverse factors: a causative brain disease, drugs used for treatment, and the psychological effect of having epilepsy with the inevitable personal, social and employment problems.

5. We are now in an age when it is appreciated that many patients with epilepsy suffer from complex partial seizures, with involvement of the temporal lobe and associated parts of the brain, which are concerned with such complex functions as memory, learning and emotions. It seems possible that these patients may have to cope with problems particular to this form of epilepsy, as well as with the more general problem of having recurrent seizures about which we will write later (p. 119).

It is hardly possible to quantify or measure personality and so to define what is meant by a normal or abnormal personality. Personality is really a social judgement. Someone able to adapt successfully to the environment in which he lives is judged as having a normal personality, but such normality depends not only on the person but also on the environment. An eccentric professor flourishing in the cloisters of an ancient university is a character. A quiet and intelligent young man thrown into the milieu of a barracks full of conscripts is a misfit: does he have a personality disorder? Adaptation to environment is a matter of learning social skills, acquiring social competence, and depends on the ability of the person and the difficulties in his environment. Let us consider how some people with epilepsy may fail in their adaptation. There are two important corollaries which follow from the proposition that personality problems are due to a failure to learn to adapt. Firstly, they are more liable to develop in those whose epilepsy started at an early age; and, secondly, they can be prevented or at least alleviated by education in social skills and by improving the environment—they are not the inevitable consequence of having epilepsy.

The ability of the patient

1. A patient with a significant degree of brain damage from an early age is likely to have a measure of intellectual impairment which will make learning more difficult, but not impossible.
2. If seizures are not controlled, the resulting brain disturbance may impair learning further.
3. Excessive or inappropriate treatment with antiepileptic drugs will affect seriously a patient's ability to cope with his environment.
4. Damage to deeply placed parts of the temporal lobes, such as may occur in small children who have uncontrolled febrile convulsions (p. 152), may impair the proper emotional reactions to learning new experiences.

The adverse effects of environment

The psychological and social problems particular to epilepsy are considered fully in Chapter 7. They contribute a part of the adverse environment with which the patient with the disadvantages mentioned above has to try to cope. Other problems, not particular to epilepsy, add to environmental stresses:
1. A poor social, economic or intellectual family background.
2. A local environment of social deprivation where housing is difficult to get and unemployment levels are high.

Problems more particular to epilepsy include:
3. The family attitude to the patient which may be one of rejection or domination and over-protection: or both.
4. Teasing, bullying, and social rejection at school are all too common, but the school and the family offer at worst a measure of security.
5. The adolescent, quite possibly rather backward and immature, faces much greater difficulties when he leaves school. He is unlikely to be able to find security and companionship in a job. At home and unemployed he will be stressed even

more by faulty parental attitudes. At an age when his sexual awareness is aroused, increasingly he will be frustrated by his failures in the mating game.

We have suggested that the development of a normal personality depends on the ability of an individual to adapt to an environment with which he can cope. We have outlined some of the disadvantages which may face the person with epilepsy. However, adaptation, successful or not, depends on the all important interaction between the individual and the environment. If there is no such interaction, there is no opportunity for adaptation. All too often the patient who becomes isolated from environmental stresses, has little opportunity for essential interactions. Perhaps, overprotected by his family, he will not be exposed to normal sanctions for his misdeeds: 'Well you see he has epilepsy'. Whether at school or in later adolescence, isolated from his peers, he has no incentive to conform to their mores: to become a 'normal personality'. Stones exposed to the buffetting of a rapid stream, soon become round and smooth: stones with an acceptably normal 'stone-personality'. Possibly stones lying for hundreds years in a stagnant pool, with sharp edges and encrustations, would be described by petrologists as exhibiting a typical 'personality of the stone'.

To return to our original three propositions. There are many reasons why some people with epilepsy should present with personality problems. This personality is not specific, but depends on the individual's disadvantages, and the particular and general stresses to which he is subject. However, much more importantly, if the problems are understood, there is much that can be done to alleviate them. The concept of the Epileptic Personality can surely be exorcized. Some patients may continue to have some personality difficulties, even with the best possible management, but then so do we all.

6

Psychological and psychiatric disturbances

We considered personality separately in Chapter 5 because of the past definition and lingering myth that there was a specific Epileptic Personality. Fortunately, there is no suggestion that people with epilepsy are necessarily mad, nor that, if they do have psychological problems, there is any psychiatric disturbance characteristic of epilepsy. In this chapter we will discuss that very wide range of psychiatric problems which patients may have to face and how they may arise.

The majority of people with epilepsy are as normal mentally as anyone else. However, as a population they do show a significantly greater incidence of psychiatric disorders. It is difficult to say just how much greater—and the statistics do not really matter much—because published reports have been weighted by groups of patients selected because they needed to be referred to general or psychiatric hospitals.

These psychological and psychiatric disturbances can be divided under three headings:

1. those related directly to the seizure: before, during or after
2. those due to the brain damage which contributed to causing epilepsy
3. those due to adverse environment factors.

Disturbances related directly to a seizure

Some of these are experienced by the patient and may cause him distress. Others are only apparent to the observer because the patient is not sufficiently conscious to record and later report what he has felt. It is quite possible that during a complex partial seizure a patient may have an experience (which is usually unpleasant) which he is not conscious enough to remember except as an overall feeling of distress. Such feelings may well have an important influence on his attitude to his seizures.

a. Before the seizure. Mood changes are quite common (p. 36) and they may give quite a useful warning* to the patient of an impending seizure. If these mood changes consistently precede a seizure, and can be identified by an intelligent patient, it should be possible to abort the attack with one of the newer rapidly acting antiepileptic drugs. The family observer can also help in this identification, and he needs to be ready to react sympathetically to transient irritability or inappropriate exuberance.

b. During the seizure. Except during complex partial seizures, the patient is unlikely to have distressing or confusing experiences, nor is the observer likely to consider the seizure as other than a physical event. We have already described some of the patient's experiences during the state of alteration of consciousness (p. 41). Not only may he live through a nightmarish world of inexplicable anxiety, fear, sense of obscenity, or even horror, but because he cannot understand, he may become convinced that he is going mad. He can be helped a great deal by discussion and explanation of the nature of his attacks. Some patients have been reassured by being shown the EEG changes during one of their seizures. The EEG record may be difficult to understand, but at least the event is there on paper, it is real, not the unreality of insanity.

Mr R was a pleasant young man in his late 20s who had moved recently into the area. He was attending the Epilepsy Clinic for the first time. He worked as a clerk in the offices of the Law Court, a job which he enjoyed and found satisfying. He had been married for four

---

* These changes may be hours or even a day or two before the seizure and are quite distinct from the aura which is the early part of a partial seizure before consciousness is affected.

years. His wife worked as a secretary and they had decided not to have a family, as there were lingering doubts about passing on epilepsy. They were both content with their work and each other.

Mr R was used to attending hospital. For past 10 or so years he had reported every six months and had been seen by an ever changing population of junior doctors. His visits were usually brief and he did not really understand why he went. His fits were quite mild and did not happen all that often. His modest dose of carbamazepine had not been changed for ages. His epilepsy was not much of a disability, but he had a problem which was worrying him more and more. He could not talk about it to his wife and there never seemed to be an occasion to discuss it with the hospital doctors. He thought he was going mad.

He suffered from complex partial seizures which had never developed to a convulsion after he had started treatment. The attacks always followed the same pattern. He seemed to be in a trance-like state. He was transfixed. To a degree he was aware of his surroundings, but he could not respond to them, and they seemed to change in a shimmering sort of way: to become dim and then suddenly very bright, to go far far away and then suddenly enlarge so that he felt Lilliputian in an enormous world. As a small child he had had an anaesthetic when his tonsils were removed. It was rather like that, or perhaps more like some nightmarish dream. There was a pervading feeling of fear. Fear not of what might happen to him, but rather of his inability to control what was happening.

Just before Mr R was due to see the consultant in the Epilepsy Clinic he had an EEG test. Perhaps he was tensed up and fussed. At any rate he had one of his typical attacks during the examination. He was really worried and he made up his mind. He would discuss his fears. After all he was seeing a consultant for the first time in years and he, if anyone, should be able to help. Indeed the consultant was most sympathetic and understanding. Realising that Mr R was an intelligent young man, he explained all about complex partial seizures and the functions of the parts of the brain involved. Mr R was relieved to have the chance to talk things over, but he was not convinced.

'Really you should not worry too much about these attacks. You don't have them very often. From your notes it seems that the last one was 6 months ago.'

'Oh, but I had one half an hour ago when I was having the EEG done.'

'Let's have a look at it and see what happened.'

The consultant and Mr R went through the EEG record together. Sure enough, during the 2 minutes or so that the attack lasted, there were obvious changes in the pattern, apparent even to Mr R.

'Thank you, doctor. Now I know that my attacks are real. I am not going mad. I have never felt so relieved in my life.'

Comment

The message of this story is obvious. Our only comment is that if patients are to make regular visits to hospital clinics such visits should serve a useful purpose. Frequent brief interviews with junior doctors overload the hospital service and are seldom useful. Occasional discussions with specialists often are.

Perhaps now that Mr R has recovered his 'sanity' he and his wife may revise their ideas about having a family.

The observer may well find the patient's behaviour during an attack extremely difficult to understand, but it should be much easier for him to accept an adequate explanation provided that this is given to him. It is worth re-emphasizing that seldom, if ever, does a patient during a complex partial seizure show meaningful violence. He is not dangerous.

Mr C, now middle aged, had been in a long-stay unit for people with epilepsy for a long time. He was popular with patients and staff because of his pleasant personality and his reputation as a hard worker, but above all his 'fits' were notorious. No one really knew how they started. The beginning was lost in the later drama. For many they were the highlight of a rather humdrum life.

Everyone knew what to do. Whenever Mr C started one of his attacks, all those near were expected to join forces to hold him down, sit on him and restrain him. Nice as he was, he was dangerous. The greater the number of helpers, the stronger he seemed to become, and the wilder and more bizarre his seizures.

A new doctor with new ideas was appointed to the unit. Staff were sceptical. He might think he knew about epilepsy but he did not understand their patients. He decreed a new policy for Mr C. When he seemed to be starting an attack he was to be left quite alone: no efforts at restraint, no audience. Mr C, who was more worried and frightened than anyone else, was told what to expect. The nursing staff accepted the new instructions, but, grimly critical, predicted severe injury to the patient and to the furniture.

After supper, some days later, most of the patients were relaxing in their sitting room in front of the TV. Mr C came in. Clearly he was not himself and even more clearly he was going to have a fit. Quietly, the others left the room. Someone turned off and unplugged the TV. They waited outside and listened anxiously. The nurse on duty discreetly looked through a communicating window.

Mr C was moving round the room picking things up and putting them down again. He took three books off the shelf and put them very carefully on the floor in front of the door. Several times he shook his head as if to clear something away. He was very pale. Suddenly he flushed and half fell, half sat on the nearest arm chair, almost collapsed. He unzipped his trousers, and then zipped them up again. He seemed to fall asleep.

Some 10 minutes later he woke up, looked around very puzzled, and left the room. He returned to his friends and wanted to know what had happened and why they had gone away. He had survived one of his attacks and all he had was a bit of a headache. The TV worked all right as soon as someone remembered to plug it in again.

The staff were confounded, the doctor was relieved, but no one was more relieved than Mr C. He was not dangerous.

A serial (or pseudo-status) absence or a complex partial seizure (p. 46) may appear to an observer as a psychiatric upset. However, they are uncommon and it is possible to identify them because there is alteration of consciousness and confusion.

c. After the seizure. The patient will be unaware of what has happened and so will not be worried, except on those occasions when he has had a prolonged period after an attack when he was unable to register memories and there seemed to have been a gap in his life. He will need explanation and reassurance. It is easier to accept inappropriate behaviour during a seizure than normal behaviour after, which he cannot recall. He may well feel that he has gone mad.

Three points need to be explained to the observer.

(i) Some complex partial seizures are very slight and may be missed, but they can be followed by several minutes of strange behaviour which is superficially sensible but over which the patient has no control. This behaviour sometimes causes legal problems (p. 139).

Mr B was a tall, heavily built man of 40. He walked slowly, he talked slowly and he seemed to think even more slowly. He had lived with his parents and had never been employed. He had frequent tonic-clonic convulsions. About 10 years before, his parents found that they were too old and infirm to deal physically with Mr B's seizures. The Social Work Department arranged for him to be looked after as a long term resident in a Centre for Epilepsy. There he did simple work in the joiner's shop. Occupation and small adjustments in his treatment caused a great improvement in his epilepsy. He had very rare convulsions and most of his attacks were slight complex partial seizures in the form of complex absences (p. 42) followed by a few minutes of confusion and altered consciousness.

He tended to keep to himself because he was not popular with the other residents. At one time they had been afraid of him as he had had a reputation for being dangerous. Since people had been warned to keep away from him when he went 'strange,' there had been no more violent outbursts. They were still a bit afraid of him because they could not understand the strange things that he did. So now they kept away from him all the time. At the worst he was mad, at the best he was not quite like other people. They remembered the time when he went out to work through the front door. Everyone knew that you used the back door when you were in working clothes. Mr B himself had done so for 10 years. Even stranger was his arrival at work with the new front door mat rolled up under his arm. And then there was that Christmas dinner. They were all sitting at the long table with fancy hats on and just starting on the Christmas pudding. Mr B got up from his chair, ambled over to the kitchen, fetched the trolley, collected everybody's plates still laden with pudding, and wheeled them off to the pig bin. Yes, it was just as well to keep away from Mr B

Comment

Before he went to the Epilepsy Centre Mr B must have suffered from secondary tonic-clonic convulsions which arose very rapidly from complex partial seizures so slight that they passed unnoticed. They were almost certainly worse because he was cooped up with elderly parents with nothing to do. The great improvement after he went to the Centre shows the value of meaningful occupation and that it is much easier to prevent the development of complex partial seizures than it is to stop them.

(ii) Those few patients whose tonic-clonic convulsions are difficult to control, from time to time have a series of such attacks (not amounting to status epilepticus). Although they may have recovered consciousness fully, their behaviour may remain bizarre and apparently 'mad' for several days.

(iii) During the stage of partial consciousness following a seizure, any interference, however well-meaning, is liable to provoke a reaction which is misinterpreted as violence. Unless it is absolutely necessary to intervene, the patient should be left alone until he has recovered full consciousness.

Brain damage

1. Severe brain damage will cause mental handicap. A high percentage of patients in hospitals for the mentally handicapped suffer from fits which are often difficult to control.

2. There are a number of rare diseases, some of which are hereditary, which result in progressive mental deterioration and also fits. Most are manifest in early childhood but some develop later in life (for example Huntington's Chorea when there are associated abnormal movements). These unfortunate

patients are unlikely to present problems to those concerned with epilepsy since their management is that of their primary disorder.

3. A small number of patients with chronic epilepsy show a progressive intellectual deterioration. The reason for this is not clear. It does not seem to be related to the number or the severity of their seizures, and there is little evidence anyway that seizures in adults (other than severe status epilepticus) cause brain damage. The following contributory factors have been suggested:

(i) Excessive treatment with antiepileptic drugs.

(ii) Repeated head injuries resulting from seizures

(iii) Some slowly progressive brain disease, possibly conse-quent upon a relatively simple childhood virus infection. The fact that most of these patients have severely abnormal EEGs would support this suggestion.

Mr H died at the age of 52.

His parents ran the local store in a small village in the South of England. He did quite well at the village school and, when he left, he helped in his father's shop for a year or two until he found a job as a gardener: a job he was good at and which suited the rather slow pace at which he liked to work. His mother died young and so he gave up his gardening to help his father. When he was 46 his father died and the shop was sold. Times had changed and Mr H found it impossible to get a job.

When he was 11 he had had a serious illness with a high tempera-ture. He was in a semi-comatose state for several days but then seemed to make a good recovery. He was looked after in the local-hospital but the cause of the trouble was never discovered. Soon after he started to have generalized convulsions. These occurred at night and did not upset his life unduly. He was treated with very large doses of antiepileptic drugs, which did not seem to help much, but which did slow him down a bit.

At the age of 46 he was admitted to a Rehabilitation Unit in the hope that he could be helped back into employment. On admission his speech was slow and his movements were clumsy. His IQ was well above average at 120. He was still having a lot of drugs, although not as many as before. They were adjusted suitably. In view of his previous experience he worked in the gardening section where he did well and he was able to take responsibility for one of the greenhouses.

Since his admission to the Rehabilitation Unit he had few fits and as before these were always at night. He had all the possible inves-tigations to exclude any general medical or particular neurological disorder. Special x-rays had shown some slight shrivelling of his brain, and his EEGs had shown consistently a very severe and generalized abnormality.

Only six years later and shortly before his death he was in a chronic hospital. He could not stand and could only totter about with help. Although he seemed to understand what was said to him, his speech was so slurred and his thought processes so slow that any conversation was impossible. He did not know really where he was, the time, the date or the year. He sat all day slumped in his wheel chair.

Comment

After he died no post-mortem was carried out and so the cause of his deterioration will never be known. Of the possible causes mentioned above:

1. His fits were never very severe.
2. They usually happened at night and so he was not at risk of repeated head injuries.

Perhaps,

1. The early over-enthusiastic treatment with antiepileptic drugs certainly caused an important degree of intoxication, which could have resulted in permanent brain damage.
2. He had some chronic infection of his brain cells following the illness he had had when he was 11 years old. The severe EEG abnormality would suggest continuing disturbance of brain function.

Such rapid and severe deterioration is rare in those with epilepsy. It is rather commoner for there to be some measure of lesser progressive decline. Since such decline may be preventable it is important that there should be further research into possible causes. Mr H's sad story is not just 'one of those things which happens to epileptics.'

4. Unlike other parts of the body the brain is unable to replace its nerve cells when they wear out. Fortunately, we are all born with huge reserves and so it is not until very late in life that these reserves are depleted sufficiently to cause impairment of intellectual function (*dementia*). Patients who have suffered significant brain damage naturally have less reserve to fall back on and are liable to dement earlier.

5. Complex partial seizures are common and they are usually due to damage to one or other temporal lobe. The role of such lesions in causing psychiatric disturbances is not clear. Certainly it would be wrong to suggest that all patients with complex seizures are disturbed. Rather we would suggest that, because of the involvement of the temporal lobes in emotional experiences and learning, these patients are less able to cope with the adverse effects of their environment.

6. Patients with brain damage are often less able to respond normally to stress (see below) and so are more liable to have anxiety or hysterical reactions.

Adverse environmental conditions

Patients with epilepsy are as liable as anyone else to develop serious mental illness (*a psychosis*). Some people have suggested that psychoses in epilepsy are related directly either to seizures or to temporal lobe dysfunction. These suggestions have come from specialized psychiatric hospitals to which are referred a highly selected type of patient. It seems likely that there is a small group of specifically epileptic psychoses and these are of considerable academic interest. However, they are very uncommon and of little relevance to this book. Apart from the effects of drugs, the psychological disturbances affecting people with epilepsy, which result from an adverse environment, are similar to those found in the general population. They are commoner because of the greater environmental stresses to which epileptic patients are subjected.

1. Excessive doses of antiepileptic drugs are liable to cause mental disorders. In mild cases these may be little more than mild confusion, slowing down and perhaps irritability. In severe cases the patient may see things which are not there (visual hallucinations), become severely depressed, or imagine wrongly that people are plotting against him (*paranoia*). When someone, who has always been mentally normal, presents some serious psychological disturbance, this should be reported to his doctor as a potentially remediable effect of incorrect treatment.

2. Patients with epilepsy are subject to two types of stress: that due to having a chronic condition which often causes personal, social or economic disadvantage; and that due to those problems peculiar to epilepsy, which will be considered in the next chapter. We will consider some of the commoner stress reactions.

(i) Anxiety is a natural response to stress and an appropriate degree of anxiety is of value in dealing with stress. It only becomes a psychological disorder when it is excessive and impairs a person's ability to deal with the stress, or when it continues after the stress is over. It is important, therefore, not to treat anxiety when it is natural. When it is considered as abnormal, if possible the patient should be helped with general support and understanding rather than with pills. Fear of public spaces (agoraphobia) is relatively common in patients with epilepsy because they are afraid of shaming themselves by having a seizure.

(ii) A patient faced with a stress situation, with which he cannot cope, may attempt to escape from the situation by developing, unconsciously, symptoms of disease. Such a reaction is termed 'hysterical' in the psychiatric as against the lay sense of the word. A hundred years ago hysterical seizures were the vogue. Nowadays they are rare except in patients who suffer from true epileptic fits. It can be difficult to sort out the epileptic from the hysterical.

Miss Q at 17 remained innocent but not ignorant of the seamier side of life. Her family lived in the industrial north-west of England. They were very poor. Her father had not worked for years and both her brothers had lost their jobs a year ago. Miss Q was terrified of her father and not without reason. The family history was appalling: violence, alcoholism, prison, with murmurings of incest and rape. From all this she seemed to have emerged cheerfully normal. Perhaps her frequent emergency admissions to the local hospital had helped to relieve some of the home tensions. Miss Q was a 'known epileptic' and her seizures were not only very severe but often prolonged and serial. The hospital social worker was convinced that home conditions were making her epilepsy worse and she arranged for her admission to an Epilepsy Centre to assess the effect of the change to a quieter and controlled environment.

She settled into the Centre well. She was of below average intelligence but described as 'sensible'. Her fits were variable and appeared to be affected little by changes in treatment. Most were severe and some were alarming. On one occasion she stopped breathing, went very blue and was given artificial respiration. Sometimes it was noted that her attacks seemed to mimic those of other patients. The staff suggested that some of them might not be epileptic. On three occasions she had continuous ambulatory EEG recordings (p. 79), each for 48 hours. In all, during these sessions she had eight attacks, which, although they varied, were all severe. During each attack all that the EEG showed was muscle artefact. These eight attacks were not epileptic. However, it was not enough to prove that she was having feigned fits. Why was she having them? She was seen several times by an experienced psychiatrist who, like everyone else, found that, despite her background, she was 'very normal.'

The next step was to reduce her antiepileptic drugs. This was done progressively until she was on a very small dose. Finally, even this was stopped and it was replaced by dummy tablets. If anything she had fewer attacks. Unfortunately, two of the untrained nursing assistants discovered that the doctors suspected that Miss Q very probably did not have epilepsy at all. A few days later she crossed them in some way and they retaliated by accusing her of being a fraud.

The effect was catastrophic. She burst into tears, dashed out of the room, beat wildly at the window panes with her clenched fists cutting her arms quite seriously. Despite reassurance, explanation, sedation and several visits by the psychiatrist, there was no improvement. She made several suicidal gestures and one attempt which could have been serious. She had to be admitted to the local mental hospital for her own protection. She stayed there for some time before she was well enough to move to a psychiatric hostel well away from her home area. Her antiepileptic drugs were not started again and, three years later, she has still had no further fits.

Comments

1. The negative EEGs during attacks do not prove that she does not or did not suffer from epilepsy. They only show that the particular attacks during the recording were not epileptic.
2. However, in this case it seems highly probable that she never had epilepsy. She has gone for three years without either antiepileptic drugs or fits.
3. Her family problems were more than she could bear. Her seizures enabled her to escape an intolerable situation, temporarily to the hospital and later, on a longer term basis, to the Epilepsy Centre.
4. It is most improbable that she put on her seizures consciously. They were a genuine hysterical reaction.
5. Her superficial appearance of normality broke down when the protection of her epilepsy was removed finally. Her fear of her father and of being sent home was probably so great that her suicidal attempts are likely to have been genuine and dangerous. Clearly, the psychiatrists thought so since they kept her in hospital for some time.

(iii) Patients with epilepsy are particularly likely to react to the stresses of their disadvantage with depressions. These may range from 'feeling a bit down' to a truly psychotic depression. Antiepileptic drugs (see above) play an important part in causing all degrees of depression. Although some milder cases can be helped effectively with general support, there is a considerable risk of suicide and, if there is the slightest doubt, the patient should be referred at once to his doctor. The rate of successful or attempted suicide is much higher in people with epilepsy than in the general populations, and it must be remembered that these people have in their possession anti-epileptic drugs which are potentially lethal.

(iv) An unreasonable feeling that 'people are against me, people are trying to do me down' constitutes a psychotic reaction of paranoia. Although attitudes towards people with epilepsy have improved a great deal in the more developed countries, prejudice remains. Patients can be helped a great deal by the acceptance that such prejudice exists, by suggesting ways of dealing with it, and appreciating that their feeling may not be altogether unreasonable. Failure to offer this help will only consolidate the patient's anxieties and will often result in his being inaccessible to reason: to his developing a fixed paranoia which would constitute a mental disorder, and might eventually require his admission to a mental hospital.

7

Problems particular to epilepsy

A patient with poorly controlled seizures has a chronic disability and will have to face all those general problems with which disabled people have to deal. In this chapter we are concerned with various problems which are particular to epilepsy.

Medical and psychosocial interactions

There are some disorders; or disabilities; which are dominated rightly by medical management. There are others in which medical intervention is more or less incidental. In between there is a whole range of conditions in which doctors and other professional people assume varying proportions of the responsibility. For example, consider two extremes of the spectrum. A boy of 13 is involved in a motor car accident and receives multiple serious injuries. These are the primary responsibilities of surgeons and doctors who must determine management. However, when he returns home, he will need care from the district nurse. The social worker may be able to help the family with practical matters such as home aids or a temporary attendance allowance. Later when he is able to return to school his teachers will need to understand that there are limitations on his activities. At the other extreme there is a middle-aged woman who is blinded as a result of poorly controlled diabetes. Although she will still need medical supervision of her diabetes, the quality of her life will depend far more on the help which she receives from para-medical professionals.

Epilepsy is almost unique in that there is a continuing inter-action between medical and psychosocial problems. In the U.K. there is still an unfortunate division between Doctors and the Rest. Doctors tend to be more interested in the acute problems of diagnosis and the organizing of drug treatment. In those who continue to have seizures, the doctors tend to lose interest. Their cause is taken up by social workers and others, who step into the gap left by the doctors, and feel that management is their affair. Perhaps the doctors assume too little responsibility, perhaps other professions too much. Either way the patients suffer. It is because in the case of epilepsy it is so especially important for all disciplines to work together that this book was written. If we have been able to give those who are not doctors adequate and intelligible medical information, they will be able to work with doctors: not under or against them.

Figure 7.1. is somewhat complex, but then so are the inter-actions between the medical and psychosocial problems of those with epilepsy. Although some of the ideas represented in the diagram are discussed elsewhere, it is useful to summarize them.

1. Fits are due to Brain Sensitivity or Brain Damage, or, more commonly, to a combination of the two in varying proportion.

2. Fits, unless well controlled, cause Psychosocial Prob-lems: problems in adaptation to the external environment. These are diverse. Let us consider some of them through the eyes of the patient.

a. At school, unless the teacher is understanding and able to lead the other children, you may face rejection and cruel ridicule. You may have limitations but you may make great efforts. If your efforts are not appreciated, and your failure emphasized, increasingly you will become frustrated, until you begin to conform to that pattern of 'a difficult epileptic child' which the ill-informed teacher expects to find.

b. You may find yourself at the bottom of the employment queue and suffer the damage to your self-esteem of repeated failures to get a job 'with no reason given.'

c. You will meet landladies who, not altogether unreasonably, suggest that you move on because of the wet beds which follow seizures you have at night.

d. Often there will be failure to fit into your own family. You may suffer quite serious psychological disturbance because you do not know where you are with those to whom you would turn for support and understanding: at one time rejected, at another overwhelmed by protection which you do not feel that you need.

e. If you had problems as a child, these are likely to be much greater when you leave the relative security and structured life of school. If your seizures are difficult to control, you may well have had a degree of brain damage, which will have made it more difficult to adapt and learn ordinary social skills; you are a bit immature. Progressively you will lose contact with your school companions, whether your friends or your persecutors. As they find jobs and later marry, increasingly you will feel isolated. At an age when you are becoming aware of sex, you will find it difficult to get a girl/boy friend because still existing prejudice will put you at the bottom of the list. Your lack of social skills will only add to your difficulties. Nowadays, so many young people have access to motor cars, an important asset in the 'mating game.' You cannot drive and it is so easy to build up a deep resentment, that this is the cause of all your problems. You may have had family problems as a child, but at least you were going to school, your day was planned. After school days, with no job and fewer and fewer friends, you are hanging about at home aimless, you get under everyone's feet: the family is all too liable to reject you even more, rather than offer the support which you need so badly.

3. People faced with the psychosocial problems which we have described are liable to react to their frustrations and psychological stresses with what can be described broadly as Behaviour Problems: that is to say behaviour which is not really acceptable to those among whom they live. It is not practicable to list these problems since they depend on the

individual and the stresses in his environment. They include reactions such as irritability, egocentricity with failure even to consider the effect of actions on other people, attention seeking when it is better to be noticed because you are bad than isolated and ignored, and suspiciousness which may start as a more or less reasonable response to hostility, but develop to a fixed attitude of suspicion which is irrational, because evidence that it is ill-founded will not be accepted (the psychosis of paranoia).

4. Not only is Brain Damage a factor in causing fits, but it makes it more difficult to deal with Psychosocial Problems and more likely that Behavioural Problems will develop.

5. Nearly all patients with continuing Fits will need treatment with Antiepileptic Drugs. If these are prescribed properly with the minimum necessary dose and the minimum number of different drugs, secondary problems are not likely to be important. However, all too often this is not the case and the drugs, which should be beneficial, increase both the Psychosocial and the Behavioural Problems.

It is worth noting that in the diagram Behavioural Problems, which have something although not much in common with the myth of the Epileptic Personality, are represented as the result of Psychosocial Problems, Brain Damage, and improper use of Antiepileptic Drugs. There is no direct connection shown between Fits and Behavioural Problems.

The five effects discussed above are the primary ones. If they were the whole story, they would not represent any problems particular to epilepsy. Doctors would do their best to deal with the problems of Brain Damage, Fits, the proper use of Antiepileptic Drugs, and Psychiatrists might on occasion be called in to cope with Behavioural Prooblems which got out of control.

It is the secondary effects, the interactions, which represent one of the problems particular to epilepsy, and which makes the co-operation of different disciplines so important.

6. Not suprisingly the Behavioural Problems mentioned will increase a patient's Psychosocial Problems.

7. However, the really significant interaction is that between Psychosocial Problems and Fits. We may not know much about the proximate precipitant of seizures, but there is no doubt that patients faced with distressing Psychosocial

Problems will have more fits, and that, if these problems can be alleviated, their Fits will get better.

8. If, because of these interactions, Fits increase, there is a very serious danger that there will be pressure on doctors, from patients, their families or others concerned, to 'do something about the Fits.' Unless the doctor is experienced, or sensible enough to seek experienced advice, the response may well be to increase the dose or add another drug. This is liable to add further to the Psychosocial and Behavioural Problems, but it is liable also actually to make the Fits worse. There is good evidence that excessive doses of Antiepileptic Drugs, or too many different drugs, not only increase fits but also produce a condition of drug intoxication when the patient is likely to confuse the issue further by reacting with attacks which are not epileptic.

Unless there is proper medical and paramedical management, there is a very real risk that a vicious cycle will develop to the point when the patient becomes a social casualty.

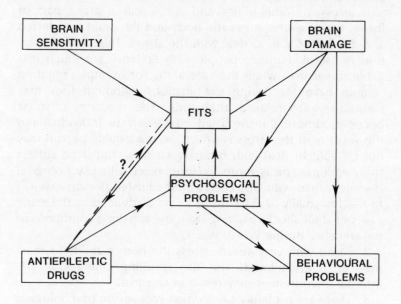

Fig. 7.1 A schema to suggest the interactions between medical and psychosocial problems. Note that it is suggested that behavioural problems are not the direct result of fits but rather of psychosocial problems, brain damage, and antiepileptic drugs.

In Chapter 3 we emphasized that epilepsy was not a diagnosis of 'doom and disaster.' The picture which we have just drawn does not contradict this principle. It applies only to those few people with epilepsy who have continuing seizures which are difficult to control. Nonetheless the interaction of medical and the psychosocial problems applies to all patients with continuing fits even if their difficulties are less severe: if they are merely disadvantaged and not disabled.

Stress

In Chapter 5, we considered stress in relation to the development of personality problems, in Chapter 6, stress as a factor in the causation of psychological disturbances, and earlier in this chapter we emphasized the importance of Psychosocial Problems in making Fits worse. There are many different types and degrees of stress and it is useful to review the general relationship between stress and seizures and the advice which should be given to patients.

1. Stresses, some minor and some major, are a part of living. Faced with a stress the body and the brain are alerted and are better able to deal with the stress. This normal reaction is useful. Further, people with epilepsy are much less liable to seizures when they are alert. For example, children seldom have fits during examinations, although they may when they are relaxed afterwards. The reaction to stress becomes abnormal if the balance between the individual and the severity of the stress is upset. An inadequate person may not be able to deal with ordinary stresses, but if he suffers from epilepsy, he is more likely to react with psychological disorders than with fits. Even a well-adjusted person may fail to react normally to extreme stress, as evidenced by the many cases of shell-shock resulting from the appalling conditions in the trenches during World War I.

2. Faced with very severe stress the body's ability to react may be overwhelmed, and the resulting changes in the internal environment may result in seizures.

3. There are probably cases when very severe psychological stress—say, the death of someone very close under unexpected and particularly distressing circumstances—may

precipitate a genuine epileptic fit, the first and perhaps the only one. It is doubtful whether this constitutes epilepsy.

4. If there is a long-term build up of the multiple stresses of the Psychosocial Problems we have referred to, if the patient is vulnerable because of a degree of brain damage, if there is no single problem with which he can deal, he may well give up. Rather than reacting to stress he will withdraw into a state of vegetative hopelessness. The increase in Fits under these conditions is due not so much to the stresses as to the lethargy, the very opposite of the alertness of the normal reaction to stress.

How then should patients be advised?

a. It is only sensible to suggest that those with epilepsy—as anyone else—should avoid excessive stress. In the case of epilepsy this is the more important because of the effect that the internal environment may have on seizures.

b. It is essential that patients should not be protected from ordinary stresses with which it is within their competence to deal. There may be those so brain-damaged that they will never be able to live ordinary lives and they will need to live in a protected environment. However, as we emphasized in Chapter 4, the great majority of those with epilepsy will find this diagnosis a minor disadvantage and not a disability. At school or in the home they must be allowed to be subject to normal stresses and disciplines. If under such conditions of intelligent care, family love and support, they cannot be helped to cope with ordinary stresses, they will never have another chance. A normal person is one who can live in a world where there are normal stresses with which he has learnt to cope. Those, and this includes doctors, who say: 'You must not upset Willie, you know he is 'an epileptic', are denying Willie the opportunity of learning to live an ordinary life. With the best intentions they are ensuring that a minor disadvantage will become a life-long disability.

Bill was 11 years old when he had his first fit. As they watched him convulsing on the dining room floor, his parents were convinced that he was dying. In the agonizingly long interval between the last jerking movement and the first deep breath back to normality, they were certain that he was dead. Bill was to have a number of attacks, and whether or not they were aware of it, those fears were always there in the back of their minds.

Their family doctor confirmed the diagnosis. There was no need for reference to hospital. He spent a long time telling the parents all about epilepsy. If he was not very reassuring at least he was very kind. As they left his surgery his final words were: 'Take great care not to upset the lad, you don't want to bring on one of his attacks.' They accepted his advice without question.

Bill was not worried by his fits. He had never witnessed one and only knew that he had had one because he had a slight headache and felt a bit achey. On the contrary, being an intelligent boy, it was not long before he realized that there were distinct advantages in having epilepsy. No longer was he forced to do any of his household chores. The flimsiest excuse let him off. He had always had frequent rows with his younger brother and sister, who irritated him. Now he could indulge his irritations: it was they who got punished. Even at school life was much easier. There was no comeback when his homework was not handed in on time. Careless and untidy work was accepted without comment.

Apparently immune from sanctions Bill became increasingly irresponsible. He found he could manipulate people and situations, he found his new power rather fun. He did not realise that he was becoming increasingly unpopular. Other children came to play, but not with him. His parents felt that the strain of 'living with epilepsy' was beginning to tell on them. Perhaps, this was what epilepsy was all about. The doctor had introduced the diagnosis in a subdued, almost sepulchral voice.

The parents talked it over many times. The father began to have his doubts. Were they tackling Bill in the right way? The mother was not so sure. The father felt that Bill should be treated a bit more like the other children. The mother repeated the doctor's final warning. One evening Bill was reminded to clean his shoes ready for school the next day. He was told to do them at once because friends were coming to supper. Bill made it quite clear that he didn't want to clean his shoes, now or ever. The father insisted. The mother was in the kitchen preparing the supper. Bill made no move to clean his shoes. The father insisted again. Bill had his fit. Did the mother say: 'I told you so?' We do not know. The father stormed out of the house: frustrated. Bill recovered quickly from his fit. He had plenty of time to clean his shoes, but he didn't. Next morning his shoes were clean and ready for him to go to school. The father had cleaned them at midnight after the guests had left.

Six years later Bill—referred to by some behind his back as 'That Bloody Willie'—was having more and more seizures in a special unit for delinquent adolescents with epilepsy. The parents were both on tranquillizers and quite uncertain how to steer their normal younger children through the perils of early adolescence. Was epilepsy, after all, a diagnosis of doom and disaster?

Comment

Did the kindly family doctor say: 'I told you so,' or should we say to the kindly family doctor: 'We could have told you so?'

Popular prejudice

There is no doubt that there is much less prejudice against epilepsy than there used to be. It is difficult to assess how much remains. There is probably little overt but quite a pool of latent prejudice. An intelligent woman presented with a questionnaire to determine her attitude to epilepsy would be likely to give all the right answers. However, the same woman might well do her very best to prevent her daughter going out with a boy with epilepsy. On a less emotive level a personnel officer would deny any objection to employing someone with epilepsy, if he was suitable. Unfortunately, all too many such applicants prove 'unsuitable'. If he was pressed, the officer would be likely to say: 'Of course I don't mind, but the people on the shop floor would not accept him'. This statement is unlikely to be true.

If we accept that there is less prejudice than some patients fear but rather more than is apparent on the surface, let us consider how it arises and what can be done about it.

1. The prejudice is described as popular, not found among bigots or extremists but in the general public. Why should this be? The general public has a lot of common sense and is well known for supporting the under-dog and helping those in trouble.

a. The seizure itself is frightening and difficult to understand. The tonic-clonic convulsion is horrific to watch and the complex partial seizure may be wholly inexplicable (p. 81).

b. A seizure is entirely inconsequential. It occurs with mystifying suddenness. There is no apparent cause.

c. The population of people with epilepsy is heterogeneous and covers a very wide range of disability (Ch. 1), but, particularly in the case of major fits, it shares a common and very obvious manifestation. Without explanation it is difficult for the man in the street to distinguish the person behind the seizure. A convulsion seems to him to be a convulsion whether the patient is a severely handicapped 'village idiot' or an intelligent shop assistant.

2. Much can be done to eliminate any residual prejudice by educating the general public and a great deal of good work has been done by various national Epilepsy Associations. Unfortunately, all too often the meetings which they organize are attended mainly by those who are not prejudiced, who do not need educating. However, they help by providing these people with facts which they can pass on. The general public reflects and absorbs the attitudes of those whom they think know better: doctors, social workers, nurses and so on. Sadly, some latent prejudice lingers on among these professional groups. Perhaps this book will help to remove it.

3. However, at the end of the day prejudice can be removed more effectively by the practice of the patient than by any amount of preaching. It is helpful if he can discuss his seizure openly with those he meets at work. He can explain what may happen during one of his attacks and what help he may need. He should not bore his audience with obsessional repetition. If he can adopt a sensible matter of fact approach to his seizures, this will soon be reflected in his colleagues. He must not use his epilepsy as a crutch, an excuse for special privileges or treatment. If he loses some time at work and others have to help him out, he must be at pains to help them out whenever he can. If he is on the look out for prejudice, is scratchy and attributes any minor difficulty to being 'an epileptic', he will soon find that he provokes the prejudice which he fears.

Overprotection

It is normal and necessary for parents to protect their young, and if a child is disabled greater protection may be necessary. Poorly controlled epilepsy calls for special precautions. Protection only creates problems when it is more than circumstances require, when it is presented thoughtlessly, or when it is concerned more with the anxieties of the parents than with the needs of the child. Let us consider various aspects of overprotection.

1. Some mothers have quite ill-founded feelings of guilt because their child has epilepsy: fearing some taint in the family or the effect of a misdemeanour during pregnancy. Other parents inwardly or even openly reject their child

because of his seizures and then feel intensely guilty for having done so. They attempt to relieve their guilt by over-protection and overindulgence. A child exposed to such conflicting emotional attitudes, even though unspoken, is liable to become confused and to develop quite serious behavioural problems.

2. We have already emphasized the importance of helping a child to learn to deal with stress, rather than protecting him from it (p. 111).

Joan was 15, the youngest member of a professional family. Both her parents were doctors, her brother a barrister and her sister just finishing a very successful time at university. Although she was of average intelligence she could not compete with the rest of the family. She was not quite clear what she was going to do, but whatever it was it must be something of her own. Her tonic-clonic convulsions were well controlled with her present drug regimen, but her little attacks were not and they were a continuing source of annoyance to herself and everyone connected with her. They were always provoked by unexpected events or little stresses: answering the telephone, reading aloud in class, or demonstrating on the blackboard. Her eyelids would flutter or jerk, her eyes would turn upwards, there would be a slight alteration of consciousness, and then within half a minute or so she would recover, albeit feeling a bit tearful. She never fell and the little attacks never developed into big ones, but slight as they were they were quite disabling and she felt that they were ruining her life.

After talking it over with the specialist, Joan and her parents had a conference with her teachers. Between them they worked out a plan. Deliberately Joan was to be challenged with situations likely to provoke her jerks. It was a long process beset by many failures as well as successes. At first the situations were simple and easy. When she had shown consistently her ability to deal with minor stresses she was offered more difficult ones to face.

Now at the age of 21 it would be difficult to recognize Joan. She shares her flat with another girl and deals confidently with a whole series of boy friends. She enjoys her job as a doctor's receptionist. It is just as well that she does not have jerks whenever the telephone rings. In fact, she has not had any jerks since she left school three years ago. Her boss teases her that it would take a patient having a heart attack in the waiting room to set her jerking now.

Comment

Jerks of the type described, unlike other types of seizure, are commonly provoked by minor stresses. Joan was able to develop this immunity to her attacks because she had the support of her teachers and her intelligent family.

3. The family will need help in deciding what precautions need to be taken in any individual case. Sometimes the doctor will provide this, but it is often more helpful for him to give general guide lines and leave it to the practice nurse, the social worker, or others to discuss the problems with the family more fully. It is no good for the doctor, or someone else, to say 'Treat Robert like the other children', or 'Just take ordinary sensible precautions'. Someone, other than the immediate family, must accept the responsibility for drawing the line between protection and overprotection. If something goes wrong, this person can bear the responsibility: the family would find the responsibility intolerable. There must be discussion. It is not a matter of laying down rules and regulations. The family must talk through their anxieties and pose the questions to which they want answers. It is of first importance to remember that the family includes the child (or the adolescent) who is having the seizure. He is himself, more often than not, frightened by the consequences of his fits and only too anxious to accept advice about precautions which he should take. However, he must feel that he is helping to make the decisions, and that they are not being imposed on him. We all need to retain our dignity. This is especially important to a child with epilepsy whose self-esteem is threatened so often. If there is sensible discussion as between equals, the patient will understand readily the anxieties of his parents and be happy to help to mitigate them. It would be altogether wrong to forbid a teenager to go out in the evening: 'Because you might have a fit'. It would be only reasonable for the teenager to tell his parents where he was going, when he expected to be back, and to telephone if he was delayed unexpectedly. He must be prepared to protect his parents from their anxieties if he wants to avoid them overprotecting him. Parental anxieties are not limited to those whose children have epilepsy and these somewhat banal suggestions apply to all families, but there is a difference which the young person with epilepsy should be capable of understanding quite well. 11.30 pm: 'She should have been home by now, I wonder what she is up to'. 11.30 pm, the front door bell rings: 'Is it the police? Is she in the hospital again?'

16-year-old Sue just could not understand it, and she was becoming decidedly irritated and just a little worried. Her mother had always been there when she got back from school, at least until today she had. Now it was nearly six o'clock. Her father was away on business. Her older brother, unemployed, was lolling in an armchair, quite unconcerned. Her older sister had settled down to her homework. She should be doing the same because she had important exams coming up soon, but she could not settle. Where was her mother?

Sue had epilepsy with rare major fits, usually at night, and occasional partial attacks in the daytime. They were a bit of a nuisance and sometimes she grumbled about them but most of the time she pretended that she did not have attacks. She was growing up and determined that everyone should know it. Yes, she really was an adult, not a child who had to be looked after because she had fits. Just now she felt very much like a child, she wanted her mother and she was getting very worried indeed. She was always there when she got back from school.

At half past seven the front door bell rang. For the past hour and a half she had been fidgeting about, staring at her school books, getting up, wandering around, sitting down again and having another go at staring. All the time it was getting clearer, something terrible had happened to her mother. She knew exactly what would happen. They would not telephone. A policeman would call to break the news personally. He would ring the front door bell. Within seconds Sue had opened the front door to Penny, her brother's latest girlfriend.

Sue had been home from school for three and a half hours when her mother opened the front door and walked in. The release of Sue's pent up anxieties overflowed into a furious verbal assault on her mother. It was some time later when the family sat down quietly to talk it all over. For months Mrs M had asked Sue to let her know when she would be home, what she was planning to do, or where she was going, and to telephone if there was any sudden change in plan. It was only polite, and Mrs M could not help worrying about Sue's attacks. But Sue was not having any, she saw it as a threat to her independence, an attempt to babyfy her. She was not mature enough or secure enough to realize that to keep in touch as her mother had asked would have been the behaviour of an independent adult.

Comment

The occasion which we have just described had, of course, been set up by Mrs M and her two other children. It was the occasion when Sue grew up.

The lost half hour

During a seizure, experiences are not able to be appreciated and for a variable amount of time afterwards they cannot be recorded as memories, although they may be understood sufficiently for the patient to react appropriately to his environment (p. 42). This is not a problem when a patient has had a tonic-clonic convulsion and is altogether and quite obviously out of touch. The problem arises when he has had a complex partial seizure. At a certain stage he will have recovered consciousness and be able to behave normally, but he will have no recollection afterwards. He may have made practical arrangements, but later in all good faith will deny that he has made them. He may have accepted instructions and, when he fails to carry them out, he will be convinced that they were never given to him. It does not require much imagination to realize that this problem, peculiar to epilepsy, can be a serious embarrassment.

Mr R was a 35-year-old civil servant. For 10 years he had been married. His wife worked as a ward sister at the Infirmary. They lived in Edinburgh in a third floor flat of a high-class, if 90 year old, tenement within easy walking distance of their work. Mrs R was in charge of the flat and of Mr R as well as her ward. Mr R did not resent this. He suffered from complex partial seizures which might last up to 10 minutes and be followed by several minutes of confusion. However, he knew when they were coming on and he was able to retire to a quiet place where his inappropriate behaviour did not embarrass his colleagues. Nevertheless, he never knew quite when they would hit him and appreciated the support to his insecurity that he got at work and from his wife.

Two years ago they decided that they had saved up enough to be able to afford to start a family, although they would have to do without Mrs R's salary. Timothy was three months old and a bonny baby. His feeding demands had been creating tensions which all too often became frank rows. Mr R took to spending the early evenings with his friends in the pub and, as Mrs R insisted all too frequently, this did not do his fits any good. Mr R was more at home with his wife's undivided attention than with her criticism. Mrs R was lonely, isolated, and getting more and more fed up with washing nappies and baby clothes. The one thing in the world which she wanted was a washing machine. The Rs were very fond of each other and one evening, after a particularly long and fruitless argument, they stopped quite suddenly, and laughed. It was all too silly, they must start again. Mr R promised faithfully to come straight home. They would save for the washing machine.

Mr R kept to his resolution, Timothy became less demanding and they had enough saved for the washing machine. All went well, that is to say until a Friday afternoon when Timothy was nearly five months old. The telephone rang. It was the office: 'Is Mr R all right? We have not seen him since lunchtime'. Mrs R became more and more worried. By the time her husband returned at 7.00 she was so frantic that she said all sorts of things which she should not have said. When it was clear that, although not drunk, he had been drinking, she said a lot more. Mr R denied vehemently that he had been drinking. It is not on record what happened after that, but on Saturday morning they took a walk with Timothy and bought a washing machine.

On Monday morning two men struggled up three flights of stairs, rang the bell and, totally exhausted, delivered a washing machine. Mrs R resuscitated them with tea and her delight. Then she washed. In early afternoon she was feeding Timothy, happily, when the door bell rang. Two more men, who were totally exhausted, delivered a washing machine.

Comment

During the Friday lunch break Mr R had had quite a severe complex partial seizure and during his confused period he had left the office and gone for a walk to clear his head. On recovering full consciousness, he had acted quite normally. He fulfilled their decision to buy a washing machine. Perhaps, he celebrated with a pint of beer. He had of course no memory of what had happened and was quite honest when he said that he had not been drinking. The memory of the pint had not registered any more than that of buying the washing machine.

It is not recorded how the second washing machine got down three flights of stairs.

Seized by the seizure

A few patients have feelings for some time before their fits (p. 36). Others are aware of the early part of their attack—the aura. They are fortunate. The majority have to live their lives, knowing that, at any time and for no predictable reason, they may be seized. Perhaps this is the greatest of the problems peculiar to epilepsy.

Not only does a patient lose contact with his environment, he loses all control of his environment. In our relationships with other people, to a degree, we all play a part. We try to present ourselves as the sort of person that we would like others to think that we are. This is not a bad thing: our ideal is likely to be an improvement on the reality. As it were, we dress up in 'psychic clothes'. These clothes help us to influence people and events. They give us room for manoeuvre, they are the subtleties of our social skills.

The patient seized by a tonic-clonic convulsion risks injury and the interruption of his affairs. The patient seized by a complex partial seizure is in a worse case. He is not convulsing on the floor. He is not someone obviously in need of help. He seems to be going about his business but he has lost all control of and responsibility for his actions. He stands 'naked' without his psychic clothes. Some people find the prospect of this unpredictable exposure a serious disability, and one which vitiates their inter-personal relationships.

The von Zs lived in North London, perhaps just a little too far North, but not so far North that the 'von' would not be appreciated. Now both in late middle age, some ten years before they had moved imperceptibly into their modest cottage with its delightful garden. They were known to everyone and they had many good acquaintances: that is everyone knew Mrs von Z at the Bridge Club and the Horticultural Society. Mr von Z remained aloof; invariably polite and courteous, he would go on regular shopping expeditions, and, of course, to the library where he ordered books not usually in demand. Everyone realised that they did not have much money, but their cottage was full of treasures from the past. To the locals they were still People of Importance. No one knew that Mr von Z suffered from complex partial seizures: few would have known what they were. Anyway, now he was getting older, he was having few attacks. Soon he should be able to get back his driving licence and he would forget about the whole thing.

Mrs von Z had finished the washing up. It was a lovely day and she went out into the garden. Mr von Z had gone off to the library. She stopped the motor mower to empty the grass box, and then she heard the telephone. Miss B, the librarian, was distraught and it was difficult to make out what she was saying. 'Mr von Z has gone mad. He tried to rape me.'

By the time she reached the library the worst of the panic was over. Her husband was sitting hunched up, alone, pale and very shaken. Miss B also was sitting alone looking pale and very shaken. At the far end of the room the local doctor was trying to explain things to the local policeman against opposition from a group of local experts. It did not take Mrs van Z long to find out what had happened. When he had handed in his books, Mr von Z had been his usual charming self. He had smiled at the young librarian and patted her arm. She was a favourite of his. Some minutes later she was startled to feel an arm round her waist. Mr von Z was at her side of the counter, trying to kiss her. He looked flushed, his eyes were glazed and his trousers were undone. In the event she had had little difficulty in avoiding the advances. Mr von Z had appeared to lose interest and had wandered off aimlessly to sit in a corner. Miss B was now shamefaced that she had panicked and rushed to the telephone. The doctor had told her about the attack which Mr von Z had had and how he would not have known what he was doing for a few minutes afterwards. It was not long before a general attitude of shamefacedness spread through the neighbourhood. Everyone tried hard to be kind and was more than understanding which was the last thing that Mr von Z wanted. He wanted his psychic clothes back again.

Comment

Mr and Mrs von Z moved and settled in a small village near Cambridge, as Mr and Mrs Z.

Although young children have not acquired much of a wardrobe of psychic clothes, the same undressing, the sudden psychological effect of being seized, is an important reason why those, who have had frequent fits from an early age, often fail to acquire those social skills so essential for normal adaptation and behaviour in later life.

8

Drug treatment

Trespassers will be persecuted

The right of complete freedom to prescribe whatever drugs they choose is guarded jealously by doctors: it is their Private Property. Probably it is wise that they should protect this property. Although in the U.K. nearly all drugs are paid for by the State, any move to suggest that the body which pays the price should call the tune is resisted most strongly in the interests of professional freedom and, we would hope, of the patient. If a GP sends his patient to hospital, he abrogates this right to the hospital doctors. If he refers a patient to a consultant for an opinion as an outpatient, it is an opinion, a recommendation, which he gets back. It is for the GP to decide whether or not to accept the advice which he is given.

It is important to emphasize this, since, if specialists have to tread with care, other advisers have to walk on eggs. Over the past decade or so, no wonder drugs have appeared to control epilepsy, but there has been a very great increase in the understanding of the way in which existing drugs should be used. Most neurologists or paediatricians and psychiatrists with an interest in epilepsy are well aware of recent advances. Many GPs and other consultants may not be. Continuing seizures cause a sense of desperation to patients and their families and there is a natural tendency to look anywhere for help, for a solution to a problem which may or may not be soluble. If you are called upon to help, you may have a very difficult decision to make: whether to advise against unnecessary and frustrating 'shopping around' or whether to suggest that it might be useful to ask the GP to refer for another opinion. The decision will depend much on the individual case: the type of patient and the quality of the GP or the present consultant. The decision you make will be determined by common sense. This chapter is not written to suggest that you should learn to write prescriptions for drugs, but rather to give you enough medical background so that you can exercise your common sense.

General principles

1. The body treats nearly all drugs as foreign substances and takes steps to get rid of them, however useful they may be. Usually this involves changing the drug chemically so that it is eliminated more easily. Most of these changes (*metabolism*) are carried out in the liver. The way in which antiepileptic drugs are metabolized is of practical importance.

a. The more quickly a drug is eliminated the more often it has to be given. Most antiepileptic drugs are got rid of quite slowly and need be taken only once or twice a day.

b. The rate at which the liver metabolises drugs is often affected by other drugs which are taken at the same time. This drug interaction can work both ways. If the new drug slows down liver metabolism of the first, this will tend to build up in the body and the patient will become intoxicated. On the other hand, if the new drug speeds up the liver metabolism, the first drug will be got rid of more quickly and there will not be enough of it to be effective.

c. In the case of some drugs the liver can metabolise them up to a certain point but then finds it increasingly difficult to deal with further doses. The effect of this is, that whereas at first an increase in dose causes a predictable increase in the amount of the drug in the blood (serum level), later quite small increases in dose will cause a large increase in serum level, which will cause intoxication.

d. When certain drugs have been given for some time, they themselves stimulate the liver to metabolise them more quickly. The dose will need to be increased to maintain an effective serum level.

These somewhat technical points have only been worked out quite recently and not all non-specialists are aware of them. Increasingly it is being realised that it is not so much the dose of the drug which is important but the amount of the drug which is present in the blood. Further, if a patient has been stabilized on a certain dose of his antiepileptic drug, doctors have to be aware of which drugs, given for some other condition, may affect the serum level. Since drug interactions apply also to additional antiepileptic drugs, it is now modern practice to use as few different antiepileptic drugs as possible. When patients are being treated for the first time, it is usually possible to use one drug only. When they have been on several different drugs it is often much more difficult to reduce the number of drugs.

2. Most patients, whose drug regime is being organized by specialists, will have estimations of serum levels until the correct dose is achieved. There is for each drug a general range of levels within which treatment is considered as most effective. Some further points should be made.

a. The range of levels is worked out from practical experience and not from any theory. It follows that it is not a rule, but rather a guide which will need to be adjusted to individual needs.

b. Levels above the accepted range are very liable to cause intoxication, and, paradoxically, excessive levels are liable to increase epileptic fits and more importantly result in attacks which are not epileptic (p. 57).

c. Measuring serum levels is useful also to make sure that patients are taking the drugs as prescribed for them.

3. We explained in Chapter 1 that epilepsy was due to a combination of brain sensitivity and brain damage, and that whereas drugs should be able to reduce brain sensitivity, they cannot repair brain damage. It follows that simple absences and primary tonic-clonic convulsions should be relatively easy to control. Partial seizures are much more difficult to treat, but it is possible to reduce their liability to develop to secondary tonic-clonic convulsions. This applies particularly to complex partial seizures which are particularly resistant to treatment. It

is less difficult to prevent their development to major fits, and it is often important to accept treatment adequate to prevent this development, and not to prescribe excessive doses of drugs to try fruitlessly to control the partial attacks: an attempt which often only makes them worse.

Antiepileptic drugs

Drug firms spend a great deal of money developing new drugs. When they find one which is effective and has passed a test for safety, they give it a name. This is the Trade Name and applies only to the drug made by the firm which developed it. Later the drug may be given an Approved (or generic) Name. At first the drug firm has a monopoly and it can recoup some of the development costs. Later, other firms are free to manufacture the drug and give it their own Trade Name. It follows that established antiepileptic drugs will have an Approved Name and one or more Trade Names. Provided that the manufacturers are reputable the effective differences will seldom be significant. Many GPs use Trade Names which are usually easier to remember. Hospital doctors usually use Approved Names. All this can be most confusing to patients. The commonly and some less commonly used antiepileptic drugs are listed in Appendix (A) with U.K. and U.S. Trade and Approved names, and with the sizes of tablets. If patients are going to other countries they should be advised to contact their Epilepsy Association (Appendix B) to find the local names of the drugs which they are taking.

1. Ethosuximide and sodium valproate are the drugs of choice for simple absences, and there are other special treatments for uncommon types of childhood epilepsy. Otherwise the choice of drug depends as much on the effect on an individual patient as on any theoretical consideration. Some people seem to do well on those drugs which are usually considered as being less effective. It is important to be able to explain to patients that because Miss M. N. is doing well on drug Y, this does not mean that Miss O. P., whose fits are not well controlled on drug X, would do better on drug Y.

2. Phenobarbitone was the first effective antiepileptic drug. Primidone, which was introduced later, works in almost the

same way because it is converted in the body to phenobarbitone. We can consider them together. They have two very important disadvantages:

a. They are liable to cause excessive sedation and, particularly in young people, irritability.

b. Once a patient has become established on one or the other it is difficult to reduce the dose, or stop the drug, without running the risk of rebound tonic-clonic convulsions or even status epilepticus.

For these reasons, in our opinion, new patients should not be started on either drug. However, if a patient is doing well and there are no signs of the side effects, it is sensible to leave well alone.

3. Phenytoin is a valuable drug but again there are problems:

a. Side effects, which are more important for young girls, include: coarsening of the features, thickening of the gums, facial hair and acne.

b. Its metabolism is complicated in two ways:

(i) There is a wide individual variation in the rate at which it is metabolised.

(ii) Beyond a certain dose the liver begins to metabolise much more slowly (1c, p. 123).

These two points are shown diagrammatically in Figure 8.1. Patient A is a rapid metaboliser, patient B a slow one, but each show a sudden rise in serum level with a small increase in dose. Ideally phenytoin should be used only when it is possible to estimate serum levels.

4. Carbamazepine is another very valuable drug, which it has been suggested is of especial use for complex partial seizures. It is helpful to be able to measure serum levels, since it tends to stimulate its own metabolism (1d, p. 123).

5. Sodium valproate, a comparatively recent drug, is of value in Primary Generalized Seizures—simple absences and primary tonic-clonic convulsions. It seems to have a particular effect on reducing Brain Sensitivity. It is less effective in controlling partial seizures, although it may be of some value in preventing their developing to major fits.

6. Diazepam and its close relation clonazepam are very effective in controlling status epilepticus. They are absorbed rapidly, and are of use also in preventing serial fits developing

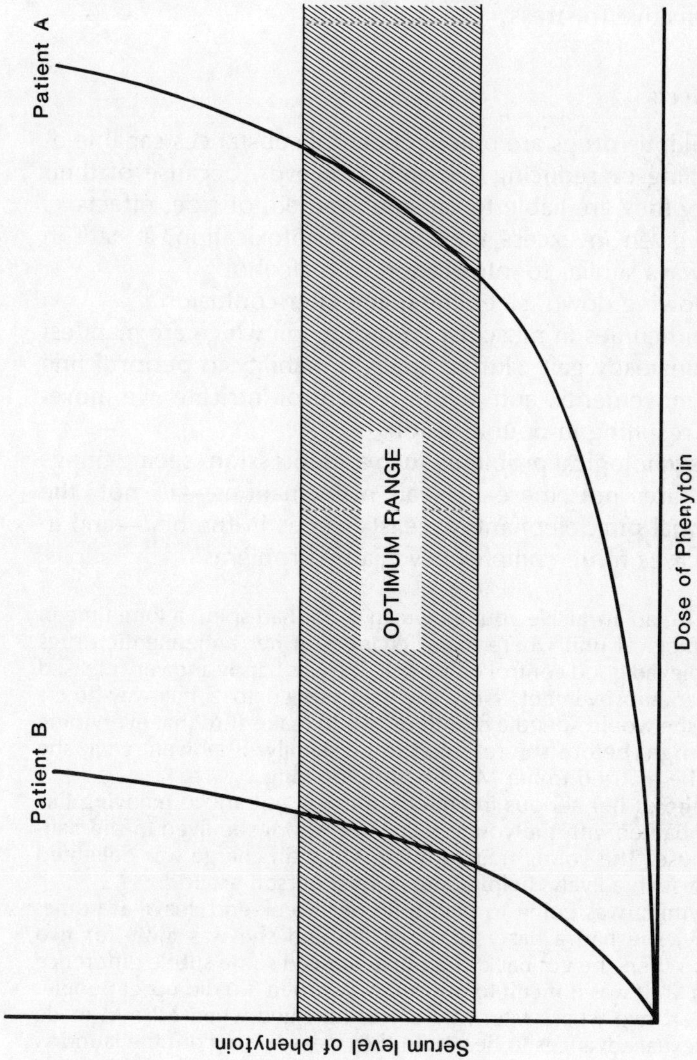

Fig. 8.1 The metabolism of phenytoin. Patient A is a rapid metabolizer and so a large dose is needed to reach the best serum level, in contrast to Patient B, who is a slow metabolizer. Beyond a certain dose the liver is unable to metabolize phenytoin quickly and so a small increase in dose results in a large increase in serum level.

to status. They are of less value if given continuously since they seem to lose their effect. However, since they are tranquillizers, they may be useful for anxious patients. Clonazepam is used for patients with 'jerks' (myoclonus) which are particularly sensitive to stress.

Side effects

Antiepileptic drugs are potent chemical substances capable of controlling or reducing seizures. However, because of their potency they are liable to cause unwanted, or side, effects.

1. If given in excess they result in intoxication, a state in many ways similar to intoxication with alcohol.

a. Slowing down, sleepiness, and later confusion.

b. Difficulties in muscular co-ordination which are manifest as an unsteady gait, slurred speech, inability to perform fine finger movements, and failure to control intricate eye movements resulting in double vision.

c. Psychological problems such as depression, seeing things which are not there (visual hallucinations)—if not the traditional pink elephants at least beetles in the bed—and in some cases more complex psychiatric problems.

Miss M, an attractive young woman of 19, had spent a long time in a neurological unit where major changes in her antiepileptic drugs had achieved good control of her fits. She was happy and very pleased with her improvement. Now she had moved to a half-way-house where she would spend a month or two to make sure that everything was all right before she returned to her family. If all went well, she would be married to her Mr O before too long.

In spite of her serious intentions she was not above enjoying flirtatious banter with the young men with whom she lived in the half-way-house. The young trained nurse Mrs C in charge was delighted to have such a lively, helpful and normal person around.

Everything was going to plan until her 'week-end' leave at home. Actually, she had a nasty attack of 'flu and she was away for two weeks. When she got back, the nurse noticed some subtle difference in Miss M. It was difficult to pin down, but then 'flu did upset people. However, two weeks later Mrs C was horrified when Miss M made overt sexual advances to her when they were sorting out the laundry.

Mrs C reported at once to the doctor in charge. He found little on his examination. There was some tremor of her hands and just a little slurring of speech. Just to make sure he took a specimen of blood, although he did not expect to find anything. She had been on a very modest dose of phenytoin ever since she had come back from the hospital and the serum level had been well within the proper range. Two days later the results came back. To everyone's surprise it showed that she was very intoxicated indeed. Miss M was questioned and she was adamant that she had been taking her tablets as prescribed. Her tablets were checked and it was apparent at once that they were twice as strong as the ones which she should have been taking (100 mg not 50 mg). The doctor telephoned her mother and it transpired that while she was on leave she had run out of tablets and her mother had used the ones which she had been taking before she went to hospital.

Back on the correct dose, after a week or so Miss M returned to her usual frivolous state. She flirted delightfully and quite innocently with the boys. Mrs C was relieved, and she and the doctor were more careful.

P.S.: Mr and Mrs O are now expecting their first baby.

Comment

The effects of intoxication are often subtle. Usually they are more or less in character, as with drunkenness, a release of inhibitions. Miss M was obviously a sexually aware young woman. Perhaps she was too fond of Mr O to approach the boys, but sufficiently uninhibited to look to Mrs C.

Because of its metabolism, intoxication with phenytoin is particularly likely to occur (p. 126).

2. Some side effects may be caused by particular drugs even in suitable doses. For example: the coarsening of the features, swelling of the gums, hairiness, and acne mentioned above as produced by phenytoin; and loss of appetite, indigestion and occasionally loss of hair as a result of sodium valproate.

3. It seems probable that even ordinary doses may cause slight effects, such as slowing down, which may be important for patients whose work involves alertness and concentration. Nowadays every effort is made to keep the dose to the minimum necessary to control seizures.

4. Often it is not appreciated that the potent antiepileptic drugs (as others) have an important effect on a patient's 'inner feelings.' If he has been stabilized on a certain drug regimen for some time he will have adapted and be unaware of these feelings. However, they will become apparent if the dose is reduced or the drug is changed. It is most important to be able to explain to the patient that his experiences are quite normal and to reassure him.

Advice to the patient

It is worthwhile summarizing this chapter by listing some of the most important points about which you should advise patients.

1. Follow the instructions which your doctor has given you. It may be dangerous to reduce the dose. To take the odd extra tablet because you are 'not feeling too good' is unlikely to make any difference.

2. If you have missed a single tablet, it does not make much difference. You can make it up next time. Most of the drugs are eliminated very slowly.

3. Report any side effects to your doctor, particularly if there has been a change in your drugs or in the dose, or if you have been given another drug for some other condition.

4. Do not press your GP to increase your drugs just because you had two attacks yesterday or one in which you were unlucky enough to hurt yourself.

5. Antiepileptic drugs are not 'drugs' like heroin or cocaine. You will need to take them for a long time but there is no danger of your becoming 'addicted.'

6. Your doctor is not a demi-God, and it would be rare to find one who thought that he was. However, if he is to help you fully, you must have full confidence in him. If you have doubts, do not just 'shop around' in the vain hope that your fits, which may be intractable to treatment, can be cured. Seek a second opinion either to restore your confidence in your GP, or that he may be advised so that this confidence may be restored.

9

Employment

People with epilepsy are at a disadvantage when looking for work. Much of this disadvantage is avoidable. Perhaps most is due to lack of information, and we hope that this book will help by providing a better understanding, but some is within the competence of the patient to overcome and in this chapter we will suggest how he may do so.

Often it is suggested that 'Epilepsy is a symptom and not a disease'. Certainly we would agree that it is not a disease, but to suggest that it is a symptom would imply that it is caused by a variety of diseases. It is more useful to consider, as we did in Chapter 1 (Fig. 1.10), that there is a wide range of the population of people with epilepsy, and that the disadvantages which accrue depend on an individual's place within the range. The problems which some people face unnecessarily are due to failure to understand this range, i.e., everyone is considered an 'epileptic'. This occurs when the person with well controlled fits, little or no brain damage, and normal intellect and behaviour, is considered just as much 'an epileptic' as the unfortunate patient with severe brain damage, significant mental handicap, and fits difficult to control; when the person with some few continuing seizures, who nevertheless has adjusted to his disadvantage and ensured that it is not a disability, is confused with that other who, unable to cope with a measure of psychosocial difficulty, presents behavioural and personality disorders (Fig. 7.1. p. 109), and in consequence is disabled.

The opportunities of ordinary employment, the arrangements for insurance and compensation for people with epilepsy, and the provision of special sheltered work for the more disabled, vary from time to time, from place to place, and from country to country. Current information is available from Employment Offices, Job Centres and local Epilepsy Associations. In the U.K., Disablement Resettlement Officers (DROs) provide a very valuable service for the more disabled, the British Epilepsy Association (p. 173) offers a useful pamphlet 'Epilepsy and Getting a Job', and the Manpower Service Commission another 'Employing Someone with Epilepsy'. We would recommend individuals to refer to these agencies. We will offer some more general advice.

The type and severity of seizures

1. People whose fits are very well controlled or who have them only at night should have little difficulty getting work. Often it is not to their advantage to register as disabled and seek the help of the DRO. Their epilepsy is not in fact a disability and they would be liable to be confused with those whom the DROs try to help: those with the disabilities of frequent fits, mental handicap or secondary personality disorders. If their nocturnal seizures are at all frequent, they would be unwise to take a job which involved an early start. At least, they should explain openly to their employer the valid reason for occasional lateness.

2. Those who consistently have a warning have an advantage. This group is likely to have complex partial seizures, which are difficult to control, but the development of which to secondary tonic-clonic seizures should have been controlled with proper treatment.

3. Simple partial seizures are not very common but those with jerking of the hands should not seek work involving delicate or expensive equipment.

4. Patients who have continuing tonic-clonic seizures despite the best possible drug treatment are likely to have significant

brain damage and some mental handicap. With some exceptions it is not sensible for them to seek open employment. They are unlikely to be successful and their failures will only prejudice employers against other less disadvantaged people with epilepsy. DROs should help them to get some form of sheltered occupation.

Tell the employer

Those registered as disabled will of course be known by their employers to be suffering from epilepsy. With few exceptions everyone else should be advised to let his employer know if he is still having seizures. The patient's doctor can be very helpful. If someone is planning to apply for a particular job, or a particular type of job, she should ask her doctor whether he feels that she can do the work adequately and safely despite her fits. If he does, he can give his patient a letter which might run something like this: 'Miss X has consulted me to ask whether I consider that in view of her epilepsy it would be suitable for her to apply for work as a . . .. In my opinion the occasional fits, which she has, should not in any way prevent her doing such work. Should you consider employing her she has given me permission to answer any questions about her epilepsy which you want to put to me. I have known Miss X for many years etc. etc.' Such a letter can be given to the employer at the stage during the interview when epilepsy is mentioned. It may well prevent immediate rejection, referral to the factory doctor who follows his rule book, or the frustrating and demoralizing: 'Thank you for coming to see me Miss X. I expect we will be writing to you.' Miss X knows only too well that they will not.

Either the applicant or his doctor should explain that the stress and anxiety of starting a new job may provoke an extra fit or two during the first few weeks. Failure to disclose epilepsy often has unfortunate results, for example:

1. If the patient is terrified of having a fit at work, he is the more likely to have one.

2. If in order to avoid having a fit at all costs, he asks his doctor for extra antiepileptic drugs, he is likely to be slowed down or intoxicated to a degree which impairs his work.

3. If he does have a fit at work, his employer might be justified in dismissing him, not because he had epilepsy but because in hiding it he was not altogether honest.

Choice of work

Obviously this will depend on local employment opportunities and on the type, severity and frequency of a person's seizures. For someone still having a significant number of fits it is important that:

1. Should he have a fit he would not be a danger to others or put himself at unacceptable risk. The employer's insurance will only cover someone with epilepsy if employed doing something suitable to his fits. However, a patient may be prepared, with his employer's permission, to take some slight personal risk in order to get a suitable job. Someone with occasional complex partial seizures should not turn down work as a grocer's assistant because he might need to use a bacon slicer from time to time.

2. If he is liable to injury in his fits he should not work in isolation.

3. He should avoid work in which the interruption caused by a fit would disrupt other people's work. Working on a production line is usually unsuitable for people having fits apart from the fact that the monotony and boredom of such work are conducive to fits.

4. He should find work within his capabilities. It is particularly important that a person with a degree of brain damage should be advised against the frustrations of unrealistic ambitions. It is often very difficult to give such advice to a previously intelligent and skilled man who, for example, suffered brain damage in a motor car accident.

Training

The person with epilepsy is at a particular disadvantage if he is looking for unskilled work. At times of unemployment he may meet prejudice and intolerance from the least educated section of the community struggling for survival. He should be encouraged to get as much training or acquire as many qualifications as possible. He should not be put off studying for fear that the strain would increase his fits. Effort and a little bit of stress are stimulating and likely to help his epilepsy. However, it is important that he should be well advised and his abilities assessed carefully, since if he tries for qualifications which are clearly beyond him, he will become demoralized and this will make his epilepsy worse.

Patients with a degree of brain damage, particularly if the temporal lobe is involved, are liable to have memory and learning difficulties. Often this makes them appear more stupid than they are. They can be trained to acquire quite complex skills provided that it is appreciated that they take longer to learn.

The people at work

It is quite common to read a report that so-and-so lost his job either because of his fits or because of the attitude of the 'other people' at work to his epilepsy. Both statements are seldom true. If so-and-so was open with his employer about his epilepsy, and if the job which he was given was considered appropriate to the seizures which he had, he is most unlikely to be fired for having seizures. More often he is kept on even if his fits become more frequent and interrupt his work quite seriously. If so-and-so loses his job the reason is much more likely to be his own fault, from which it follows that it should be within his competence to keep his job. Much the same applies to the attitudes of other people. Most other people are essentially kind and helpful, particularly to the weak and the disadvantaged. How then can so-and-so be advised so that he can keep the job which he may have had such difficulty in getting?

1. The people with whom he works are likely to reflect his own attitude to his epilepsy. If he has adjusted to it well and treats it as just one of those things, like say an attack of migraine, so will they. He should explain to those with whom he is in close contact what his fits are like and what help, if any, he needs. Almost certainly he will get it. If he has made epilepsy the extent of his experience and talks about it continuously, other people will get fed up with epilepsy and with him: it is not the centre of their world.

2. He must not allow himself to use his epilepsy as a crutch, an excuse for avoiding work or unpleasant chores. If he does

lose time and others have to cover for him, he must make every effort to make it up to them when he is able to do so.

3. Someone with continuing fits is likely to be so thankful that he has managed to get a job that he will work harder and more conscientiously than the 'other people'. Even when jobs are scarce, in all fairness they will appreciate that he deserves his.

Misemployment and unemployment

Paid employment is primarily an economic necessity, but for many people it is essential for self-respect, an opportunity for achievement. In countries which make adequate welfare provision for the unemployed these secondary considerations are often the more important. Those concerned with helping people with epilepsy to employment should beware of providing them with work at any cost: too often at the price of their personal dignity. For example:

1. A young man from a professional family, or a skilled engineer with fits from a head injury, would be misemployed as a lavatory attendant or a washer-up in a café. Neither his family nor his wife in the evening would ask: 'What sort of a day did you have?'

2. The slightly mentally handicapped son of a well-to-do factory owner would not be so mentally handicapped that he could not appreciate that the job which his father had found for him in the factory was not a real job: and everyone in the factory would appreciate it too.

Present technical advances have caused high levels of unemployment in developed countries and many able people will need to readjust from the somewhat puritanical work ethic that the only complete man is the man who is in paid employment—even if this employment is no more than tightening five nuts on the wheel of a motor car some thousand times a day. In such times the person with epilepsy who has some disadvantage will be in need of help to adjust. His situation is somewhat similar to an active healthy man of 65 who is required by regulation to retire. There is ample scope for counsellors to ensure that their lives are not 'idle and unemployed' but rather 'active and occupied usefully.'

10

Epilepsy and crime

Press Reports, May 4th 1984

Mrs A. B. (80) of 50, The Lane, North London, on her way back from Bingo last night was attacked brutally by C. D. (28) a known epileptic and all her winnings of £7.80 were taken.

Mrs E. F. (81) of 49, The Avenue, South London, on her way back from Bingo last night was attacked brutally by G. H. (29), well known to the police as suffering from chronic indigestion, and all her winnings of £7.85 were taken.

The second report is fiction. Sadly, the first is fact. For some reason the word 'epileptic' adds to the report's news value, but although it is totally irrelevant, it serves to fan the flames of the smouldering fires of prejudice. Since there is still quite a widespread belief that there is an association between epilepsy and crime—and particularly crimes of violence—and since this belief is ill-founded, it is worth considering it in some detail so that you can help to explode the myth. In parallel to the supposed association between epilepsy and crime, it is still quite common for people with epilepsy, who do commit offences, to adduce epilepsy as a mitigating factor in their defence. Seldom is this valid and when crimes are committed in relation to seizures, complex medico-legal issues arise which need to be explained.

1. Violence. There is no evidence that those with epilepsy are more or less likely to commit crimes of violence. However, some relationships between epilepsy and violent behaviour are worth summarizing.

a. Patients are liable to be violent if they are interfered with—however good the intentions—during the period of confusion and altered consciousness after a seizure (p. 98).

b. Children and young people react violently if teased and goaded by their peers. Those with epilepsy are both particularly likely to be sensitive about their fits and to be the object of childish torment.

c. A child who has suffered early brain damage often has fits and a degree of mental handicap. Because of his brain damage and the psychosocial problems consequent upon his epilepsy he will fail to adapt as he grows up, and fail to learn the social skills of inter-personal relationships. He will be liable to react to situations with which he is unable to cope by difficult or even aggressive behaviour (p. 20).

d. Phenobarbitone and primidone are known to increase irritability, particularly in young people (p. 126). Unfortunately children are still treated with these drugs which may exacerbate the difficulties of (b) and (c).

2. Petty crime. The population of those in prison for petty crimes shows an excess of those with epilepsy. This can be explained in two ways:

a. socially deprived and rejected, they are a good deal more likely to drift into minor crime

b. those with brain damage and some mental handicap are much more likely to be caught.

3. Epilepsy as an excuse for a crime with intent. It is not uncommon for a person with epilepsy, who has committed a perfectly ordinary intentional crime, to try to get off because of his epilepsy. If what he did was sensible and appropriate to the situation—although wrong—he must have been fully conscious, fully aware of his environment. Therefore, his behaviour was related in no way to a seizure and the fact that he suffered from epilepsy was no more relevant than if he had suffered from bronchitis or a stomach ulcer. The only exception would be if he was mentally handicapped as a result of brain damage, which had also caused his seizures. In this case he should base his defence on his mental handicap and not on his epilepsy.

4. *Epilepsy as a defence for a crime without intent.* However unacceptable a person's behaviour, it cannot be considered as criminal, unless he can be shown to be capable of forming the intention of doing wrong. A mentally disturbed (psychotic) patient suffering from the delusion that her husband was trying to poison her, who killed him with the kitchen knife, did not commit a crime. She would be considered as incapable of forming the intention to kill because of her mental state. She would be classified as 'Not Guilty by reason of Insanity.' She would not be imprisoned for a crime which she was incapable of committing, but, quite properly, she would be sent to a hospital for the criminally insane, at least until she was considered to be cured of her psychosis. Otherwise, she might remarry and do it again. This situation is straightforward. We are dealing with a psychosis which may be permanent or which may be present continuously for a period.

Epilepsy presents much more complex medico-legal problems since it is an episodic disorder. In relation to the seizure the patient will be in a state of altered consciousness, and so not responsible for his actions, but between seizures he is a normal and fully responsible person.

During the period of confusion following complex partial seizures a patient may commit minor offences. Perhaps he exposes himself and causes embarrassment and consternation. Perhaps he wanders into someone's garden and is suspected of loitering with intent. With adequate medical evidence and common sense such episodes should not cause difficulties. If, however, whether in such minor or in more serious cases, the patient with epilepsy does come before the Courts, what is his position? There are two possible verdicts:

a. Not Guilty by reason of insanity. He goes to a hospital for the criminally insane

b. Not Guilty by reason of non-insane automatism (actions for which he is not responsible). He is let off.

It is worth emphasizing that the primary function of the Courts (at least in civilized countries) is not to punish the miscreant but rather to protect the public. Uncontrolled epilepsy is a continuing Primary Brain Disorder (p. 9).

Consider a patient who, during a period of confusion and altered consciousness after a fit, lashed out and injured seriously someone near him. Clearly, he is not guilty of a crime since his actions were outwith his control and without intent. However, what he did was due to continuing disorder of the brain which the Law defines as insanity. 'Not Guilty by reason of insanity.' Since it might happen again he needs to be sent away in order to protect the public.

Conditions outside the brain may affect brain function (p. 5) and cause, say, seizures or periods of confusion. In as far as the causative condition can be treated, there is no continuing brain disorder and so no future danger to the public.

For example:

(i) A young person suffering from severe diabetes is being treated with large doses of insulin. He misses the main meal of the day when his car breaks down. His blood sugar falls, he becomes confused and makes a wholly unprovoked attack on the garage man who comes to help him.

(ii) A middle-aged woman becomes depressed and is prescribed one of those antidepressant drugs which may provoke seizures. She does have a tonic-clonic convulsion. As she is recovering, she attacks her husband who is doing his best to help her. It is assumed that she does not have epilepsy since, if she did not take the antidepressant, she would have no further seizures. 'Not Guilty by reason of non-insane automatism.'

Finally, a story to show that the person with epilepsy needs to be very careful about using epilepsy in his defence. A sensible man of 45 had complex partial seizures as a result of a head injury received during the war. He had complex absences (p. 42) which often passed almost unnoticed but which were followed by several minutes of altered consciousness during which his behaviour was superficially sensible but was outwith his control. One day he walked into a book shop and started to browse around. He had one of his complex absences, picked up several books, put them in his pockets without effort at concealment and left the shop. The manager stopped him, called the police and charged him with shoplifting. The case came to Court.

It was agreed that he had had a seizure, that he had not intended to steal the books, and that his offence was due to a state of altered consciousness caused by his epilepsy. If he persisted with this defence would he not be found 'Not Guilty by reason of insanity' and committed to spend the rest of his life and his war pension in a hospital for the criminally insane?

But No. On the day of the offence he had been to see his doctor who had taken a blood sample to check that the serum level of his antiepileptic drug was correct. The result came just in time. Although he showed no evidence of intoxication, his serum level was just into the intoxication range.

He was let off because it was considered possible (just) that his behaviour might have been affected by the excess of anti-epileptic drug: something which could be put right.

11

Marriage and having children

Almost invariably when someone asks advice about his plans for marriage, he is seeking confirmation of decisions he has taken already. The person with epilepsy is in no different case and his adviser, for whom we are writing, needs to be particularly circumspect because of lingering sensitivities and at the same time sufficiently informed to be able to push aside lingering myths.

To understand and advise it is necessary to remember the wide range of the population of people with epilepsy (Ch. 1). Not only is the severity of the epilepsy important, but so is the extent to which it is due to brain sensitivity or to brain damage. If brain sensitivity is the main or only cause, the patient is likely to have normal intellect and mood, his seizures are easier to control, and his epilepsy is not much of a problem. If there is an important element of brain damage, not only will his fits be more difficult to control, but he will have a degree of mental handicap, and possibly psychiatric disturbance, which will be much more disabling than his epilepsy.

Unless there is some religious bar to contraception it is possible to separate the question of marriage from the problem of whether or not to have children. There is no reason at all why a person with epilepsy should be advised against marriage just because he has epilepsy. There is no reason at all why two people with epilepsy should be advised against marriage just because they have epilepsy. There are, however, certain cautions which apply to some people with epilepsy.

Marriage: possible problems

1. If there is a significant degree of mental handicap, the patient may not be able to assume the responsibilities of marriage: whether as the wage earner or the home maker. If in addition there are seizures which are difficult to control the difficulties will be that much greater.

2. Patients having seizures are at a social disadvantage; they may be isolated by their failure to develop social skills, and objects of covert prejudice. A girl may not think twice about marrying a boy with epilepsy of whom she is fond, but her mother might well place every obstacle in her way of going out with an 'epileptic.' The great majority of ordinary marriages are between people of roughly the same cultural and intellectual backgrounds, thus making for stability. With important exceptions, if there is a marked disparity between partners, there is greater potential for instability and future problems. Patients who have initial difficulties in establishing relationships with the opposite sex should, if possible, be prevented from marrying, in their frustration, someone too much 'beneath them.'

3. There may also be a problem the other way round. A successful marriage should be a partnership in which each partner does what he does best or tries to do what his spouse does not do so well. There are some dominant people who seem to fulfill themselves by tending lame ducks. It is not unusual to find someone with epilepsy married to and supported completely by husband or wife. In this marriage there is danger of failure. The patient loses self-respect and the partner is too busy being saintly to understand.

4. Quite a high proportion of men with continuing complex partial seizures have much reduced sexual interest. Most of these will not get married at all, but, if they do, tensions may develop. Women do not seem to be affected in this way.

5. Antiepileptic drugs influence the metabolism of the contraceptive pill. Women who are taking these drugs should seek expert advice from a Family Planning Clinic.

6. There are many advantages in two people with epilepsy getting married. If they are well adjusted to their epilepsy, they can support each other and reinforce their adjustment. On the other hand, if they have problems, whether psychological or practical, their problems will be compounded and often the marriage will end in disaster.

Having children

Patients are much more likely to seek and accept advice about having a family than they are about whom they should marry! This can be divided into practical advice and information about the risk of a child having fits.

Practical problems

1. Having children involves responsibilities additional to those of getting married. The ability to assume these should be talked through and, if the couple are not very intelligent, even very obvious points need to be raised. If the husband has fits and cannot get work and his wife is the breadwinner, how will they manage when she has to give up her job? Later, will she go back to work and will her husband be willing and able to look after a small baby? If the wife has fits will she be able to look after the baby safely?

2. If the couple have decided to have a baby and if it is the wife who is having fits, she will be in a particularly receptive frame of mind for training in all those good habits which may have lapsed before. Say to her 'make sure that someone knows when you are going to have a bath.' 'Don't rely on your warning, pretend that you do not have one and avoid possible danger like standing about at the top of the stairs.' Precautions, which might seem to make a patient over-concerned with her epilepsy, are quite natural and acceptable when they are for the baby's sake.

3. Pregnancy has a variable effect on the occurrence of seizures. It is particularly important that the mother-to-be follows the instructions that her doctor has given her about drug dosage. To 'take a few extra for the sake of the baby' is likely to risk intoxication with potentially dangerous effects on the maturing foetus. Antiepileptic drugs cause a very slight

increase in the risk of congenital abnormalities. A mother, who has heard exaggerated reports of this risk, may reduce or even stop her drugs, and put both her baby and herself at very serious risk if she develops status epilepticus.

4. After the baby is born the health visitor or the district nurse can offer plenty of practical advice. If seizures are at all frequent it is sensible for the mother to look after the baby, whenever possible, on the floor, making use of mattresses, pillows and floor cushions. She should have a 'life-line' if she is not well. If there is no Granny, Auntie, or good neighbour on whom she can rely, she should be able to call on the district or practice nurse. There are still social workers who feel that a baby must be taken into care if the mother is having continuing seizures. Only under exceptional circumstances should this be necessary. Such separation would have serious emotional consequences for both mother and child and can nearly always be avoided by sensible planning. Babies grow up quickly and it is not too early to make sure that the mother's antiepileptic drugs are kept safely and well out of the child's reach.

The risk of inheritance of fits

This is a point which is raised by almost all responsible parents when one or both suffers from epilepsy. Definitive opinion should be given by the doctor, or sometimes a genetic counsellor, but others who may be asked for advice should have a general understanding of the position.

1. We have explained that people are born with varying degrees of brain sensitivity and it is probable that it is this which is inherited. It may be manifested in various ways:

a. primary generalized epilepsy either in the form of simple absences or tonic-clonic convulsions

b. febrile convulsions

c. an EEG pattern similar to that during a simple absence (p. 32) occurring either spontaneously, or as a result of provocation by overbreathing or flickering light, but without necessarily any seizures.

It follows that, if the parent has primary generalized epilepsy or a family history of EEG changes or febrile convulsions, the child is more likely to inherit increased brain sensitivity.

However, although this means that he will be more likely to have fits, it does not mean that he will.

2. If the parent's epilepsy is obviously due to some serious brain damage, for example a serious head injury, the contributory factor of brain sensitivity may well be quite slight and so the risk to the child much less.

3. There are several conditions, which are not very rare, which are strongly hereditary and in which there is brain damage which results in epilepsy. It is now appreciated that these diseases can take very minor forms, which are difficult to detect, but which may nevertheless result in seizures. If the parent has one of these minor forms, the risk to the child is high. In this case it will be necessary to go very carefully into the family history and to seek expert genetic advice.

4. If both parents suffer from epilepsy the risk to the child is considerable and most people would advise against their having children, particularly since their combined disabilities would add considerably to the practical problems.

Further points

1. Fits due to brain sensitivity are easier to control than those due to brain damage. Since it is usually the brain sensitivity element which is inherited, the prospects for the child are not too gloomy.

2. If a parent has epilepsy, there is an important increased risk of a child having febrile convulsions. If these are controlled quickly, the risk of later epilepsy is very much reduced. Parents should, therefore, get advice from their GP on how to deal urgently with febrile convulsions should they occur (p. 152).

3. If a parent has epilepsy, the child should not be immunized against whooping cough (p. 153).

4. Throughout this book we have tried to put the diagnosis of epilepsy into perspective, to cut it down to size. It is not a diagnosis of doom and disaster. A disadvantage, occasionally a significant disability, usually able to be controlled, it is compatible with normal personality and a normal life.

Mr X and Mrs X (who has fits) have thought the matter over, taken advice, and decided to have a family. If little Miss X has epilepsy this is not a disaster and above all it is not an occasion for guilt. If complicated feelings of guilt develop, if Mr X gets at Mrs X, the family will be an unhappy one. An unhappy family will be a much greater disability for Miss X than her epilepsy. If Mr X truly loved Mrs X and accepted her and her epilepsy, surely he can accept his daughter. Furthermore, surely Mrs X, who has coped successfully herself, is the best person to help her daughter to turn a disability into a minor disadvantage.

12

The young child

The form which seizures take depends on the state of maturation of the brain, and so those of the very young child will be different from those described in Chapter 2. A premature infant's brain is incapable of having tonic-clonic convulsions. His seizures are more likely to consist of odd sucking movements, irregular breathing, little jerks, or unexpected violent movements of his legs. Even up to one year typical grand mal fits are rare and attacks take the form of local or general twitching, or stiffening of the whole body with arching of the back.

In this chapter we will consider various conditions which affect the child within the first five years of life.

1. Fits provoked by conditions outside the brain

Fits are common during the first month of life. Many of these are due to brain damage before or at birth and they can only be prevented by antenatal supervision and good obstetric care. However, an important number are due to events outside the brain—abnormalities of the internal environment. It is essential that they should be recognized since they can be treated. If they are not recognized and the child is classified as 'epileptic,' he will continue to have seizures. These will damage his immature brain, resulting in mental handicap and fits in later life—he will come to suffer from epilepsy.

Some of the more important remediable conditions are:

a. *Low serum calcium.* Fits start towards the end of the first week of life and are commoner in artificially fed babies.

b. *Low blood glucose.* This is liable to be found in very small babies or those born to diabetic mothers being treated with insulin.

c. *Lack of pyridoxine* (one of the B group of vitamins) can cause fits and may be due to poor diet or an hereditary disturbance of metabolism.

d. *Sudden withdrawal of phenobarbitone* may cause seizures (p. 126). If the baby's mother has been taking phenobarbitone for epilepsy, some will have got into his blood. After birth his phenobarbitone level will fall and he may have seizures. These are easy to control. The baby has fits but he did not inherit his mother's epilepsy—only her phenobarbitone.

These problems are dealt with by the specialists in the neonatal unit, but it is useful to be able to explain to the family that such fits, which are quite easy to control, do not mean that the baby is going to suffer from epilepsy in later life.

2. Reflex attacks

Young children, usually under about four years, are liable to attacks which are somewhat like adult faints. Provoked by a sudden fright, a surprise, or perhaps a relatively minor injury, the autonomic control of either breathing or heart beat is upset and either:

a. The child stops breathing and becomes more and more blue, or

b. His heart stops for a time and he becomes suddenly very pale.

In either case, if the attack lasts long enough, the brain will be starved of oxygen, the child will lose consciousness and may have jerks which mimic a seizure. Although alarming, these attacks are not dangerous and they are not epilepsy.

3. Age-dependent reactions to severe brain damage

There are many ways in which a child may have acquired severe but non-fatal brain damage. Faulty development in the womb and certain infections of the mother during pregnancy result in the baby being born with an abnormal brain. The brain can be damaged at birth by mechanical factors, lack of oxygen, or bleeding into it. Infections of the brain or the covering meninges cause severe damage to the immature brain. There are a large number of disorders of metabolism, some of which are inherited and most of which are rare, which cause widespread damage to nerve cells throughout the brain.

Severe brain damage causes two quite different conditions depending on the age when they develop. Both are comparatively uncommon. They are difficult to treat and the majority of children develop mental retardation severe enough to require institutional care. Many, later, have various forms of epilepsy. Occasionally when there is no obvious history of brain damage the child responds to treatment and recovers. It is possible that these fortunate few had some acute and self-limiting brain disorder.

These conditions are worth mentioning briefly because of the gloomy outlook. In these cases the fits are all too often a diagnosis of doom and it would be unkind to offer the family optimistic reassurance.

a. Infantile spasms. The child is aged between 3 and 12 months. In the attacks the infant cries, his head nods and his arms and legs flex. Often termed 'salaam attacks', they come in groups with as many as 50 at a time. The movements, although sudden, are slower than jerks (myoclonus) seen in other types of fit. The EEG (Fig. 12.1) is chaotic with very high voltage slow waves and frequent spikes, suggesting severe interference with brain cell function. The attacks and the EEG abnormalities can usually be controlled with hormones—they do not respond to the ordinary antiepileptic drugs—but except in the rare cases mentioned above this does not prevent the progression to severe mental retardation.

b. Myoclonic epilepsy. The child is aged between 3 and 7 years. The characteristic seizure consists of sudden myoclonic jerks which often throw the child to the ground with serious risk of head injuries. There are often other types of seizures such as atypical absences and tonic-clonic convulsions. The best treatment is with drugs related to diazepam, but although the jerks tend to subside as the child gets older, most patients continue to have fits and become mentally retarded.

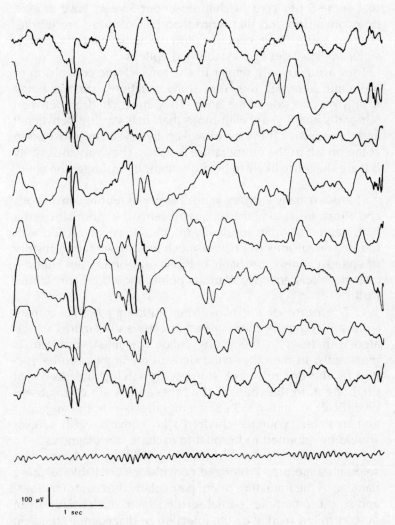

Fig. 12.1 The record from a child with infantile spasms. The whole record is disorganized with very large slow waves and frequent spikes. Contrast with the better organized abnormality in Figure 2.8. See also caption for Figure 1.1.

4. Febrile convulsions

Febrile convulsions are common and important. It is estimated that some 5 per cent of children under 5 years have at least one convulsion and that more than half of these are febrile. Further, about 10 per cent of children who have febrile convulsions will later develop established epilepsy.

They are generally similar to the tonic-clonic convulsion of the adult, although they may show variations, such as being mainly on one side of the body. They affect children between 6 months and 5 years with more than half starting between 9 and 20 months. They are provoked by fever and most often come on when the temperature is rising. They vary in severity but are the more likely to be prolonged, the younger the child.

There is usually a strong family history of febrile convulsions and it can be assumed that it represents the inheritance of a high degree of brain sensitivity (p. 19). However, a child with febrile convulsions will have a much less strong family history of epilepsy. This is probably because only one in ten children later develops epilepsy. Various points should be considered further.

a. The cause of the convulsion. Although febrile convulsions are common, there are other causes of seizures associated with fever in the young child. The most important is meningitis. In the older child signs of meningitis can be elicited by the doctor—neck stiffness, irritability and dislike of bright light. In the younger child these signs are often absent or difficult to find (p. 59). Since meningitis is both dangerous and treatable, younger children who convulse with a fever should be admitted to hospital to exclude this diagnosis.

b. Immediate treatment. Brief febrile convulsions are seldom dangerous. Prolonged convulsions are liable to cause damage to the immature brain, particularly the temporal lobes, and so cause complex partial seizures later. Such seizures can be controlled readily by the injection of diazepam into a vein (if possible) or into the back passage (rectum). If the convulsion is other than brief, a doctor must be called at once. If he is not available, the child must be taken to the nearest hospital.

If the child has already had a febrile convulsion, it is as well to instruct the mother (if she is sufficiently sensible) how to give diazepam into the rectum should the child develop a fever.

c. The risk of later epilepsy. This is relatively slight (one in ten cases) and most mothers can be reassured. The factors which increase the risk have been worked out.

(i) Severe and prolonged seizures

(ii) Early onset of the first convulsion

(iii) A history of some degree of early brain damage

(iv) A family history of epilepsy.

d. Treatment to prevent a second attack. There is no agreed policy as to whether children who have had one febrile convulsion should be given regular treatment to prevent another. There are alternatives.

(i) The mother should be instructed to treat any fever quickly with regular tepid sponging and perhaps juvenile aspirin. Possibly she might give diazepam into the rectum. At least she should be told to call the doctor immediately if there should be a convulsion.

(ii) If there are operative risk factors (see above) some doctors advise giving regular antiepileptic drugs to prevent a recurrence. Both phenobarbitone and sodium valproate have been shown to be effective. In our opinion the giving of long term antiepileptic drugs to young children with maturing brains should be avoided if possible. If it is considered necessary, sodium valproate is the drug of choice since phenobarbitone is liable to cause irritability, a general slowing down, and to impair learning and development.

5. Whooping cough immunization

Very rarely immunization against whooping cough can have disastrous consequences. The child has a severe brain disturbance which results in permanent mental retardation and epilepsy. Sometimes the brain damage is the result of prolonged status epilepticus provoked by the immunization.

In the U.K. publicity given to these unfortunate reactions has had two results.

Firstly, there has been a most unfortunate decline in the number of children being immunized—unfortunate, because taken overall the dangers of whooping cough are considerably greater than those of immunization.

Secondly, legislation has been introduced to provide generous compensation to those children whose disability can be attributed to immunization.

Although there is strong official recommendation that children should be immunized, there are two groups to whom this does not apply.

a. Those with a history of some degree of early brain damage.

b. Those with a family history of epilepsy in close relatives—brothers, sisters, parents, grandparents, uncles and aunts.

These are two of the risk factors for the development of continuing epilepsy after febrile convulsions (p. 153).

Parents should be advised that, if they have a child who is mentally retarded with epilepsy and who has been immunized, they will only qualify for compensation if it can be proved that there was a severe brain reaction—such as status epilepticus—immediately after immunization.

13

The school child

It is present theory (if not always practice) that 'whenever possible' handicapped children should be sent to ordinary schools rather than to special schools either for the handicapped or for children with their particular handicap. Unfortunately, there are many children with epilepsy due to severe brain damage, who are mentally handicapped to an extent which makes ordinary education impossible. In this chapter we will consider only children capable of going to ordinary schools, and how the medical and psychosocial interactions discussed in Chapter 7 (see also Fig. 7.1, p. 109) apply to children. Parents not only need but are ready to accept counselling to help with the many problems of the epileptic child.

Medical and psychosocial interactions in the school child

1. Seizures

These are generally similar to the adult types described in Chapter 2. There are two relevant points:

a. Primary generalized seizures start during early school years. They are comparatively uncommon and, by definition, are not associated with brain damage and mental handicap.

They do not call for detailed investigation. To carry out unnecessary investigations would distress the young child unduly, and it is important to explain to parents that they are not done because they are unnecessary, and not because the doctor is negligent. The rather rare simple absences as well as the much commoner complex absences will interfere with school work and often it is difficult for the teacher to appreciate how often they occur.

b. In adults, tonic-clonic convulsions, whether primary or secondary, should be able to be controlled well with appropriate treatment, unless there is severe brain damage. In children they are much more difficult to control. The adult may have frequent complex partial seizures which seldom generalize. The child may have frequent slight complex partial seizures in the form of complex absences, but more prolonged ones are less common because they are more likely to generalize.

2. Antiepileptic drugs

These must be used with particular care in children.

a. Phenobarbitone and the related primidone should be avoided. On the one hand, they may cause irritability and hyperactivity, and, on the other, a slowing down which impairs school performance.

b. The child is particularly sensitive to excessive doses which cause behavioural disorders and serious disruption of learning.

c. It is uncertain how far normal doses of drugs may affect the maturing brain—perhaps permanently—as it is uncertain how far continuing fits, or even electrical brain disturbance without clinical fits, may do so.

Fortunately paediatricians have a good understanding of these problems, and any child with continuing seizures should have ready access to their specialist advice.

3. Brain damage

Even a degree of brain damage unlikely to result in mental handicap, for example that in the temporal lobe following uncontrolled febrile convulsions, can cause learning difficulties.

a. In right handed people speech is controlled from the left side of the brain. If this side is affected, the child may be slow to learn to read or have difficulties in handling symbols such as numbers.

b. Right brain damage impairs the appreciation of visuo-spatial relationships.

c. The temporal lobes are associated with the emotions, and if affected, failure of the appropriate emotional reaction to the learning of new experiences can lead to behavioural problems.

4. Psychosocial problems

Apart from the medical factors which cause difficulties for the child at school, there are significant psychosocial problems which will be liable not only to exacerbate seizures but also to result in behavioural disturbances. It is significant that more children need to be excluded from ordinary schools because of their behaviour than because of their fits.

a. The family base. All too often a child with epilepsy creates an atmosphere of disruption and unease so that he is deprived of that secure home base which he needs so much to deal with his problems at school.

b. Too many teachers, without adequate understanding of the problems of the epileptic child, treat him as much more stupid than he is, and are unable to provide him with the specialized help which he needs to overcome this apparent stupidity.

c. Unless the correct attitudes (which we will consider) of the child, the teacher and the other children are established, he is at risk of the persecution and ridicule which can be offered so cruelly only by the young to the young.

If a child with poorly controlled seizures and/or significant brain damage is to be educated in ordinary schools, it is essential that special provision is made for him. The extent of his intellectual and learning difficulties should be assessed by a psychologist experienced in epilepsy and his teachers should be told how they can help him in class. It is valuable to have special residential schools for children with epilepsy. These should be used not only for the long term education of those too handicapped to attend normal schools, but also for the short term admission of those having problems at school, in order to determine the causes of their difficulties and if possible to correct them before returning to the orginal school. These schools should be centres of excellence where research is carried out and teachers trained to handle problems peculiar to the child with epilepsy. These teachers would then be available to visit schools throughout the country to instruct and supervise teachers with epileptic children.

If proper provision is not made for these children they will become bored and frustrated in school and, in consequence, their fits will get worse and their behaviour will deteriorate. A vicious cycle develops: more fits, more drugs; more drugs, more learning and behavioural problems; more behavioural problems, more problems at school: and so on. It is not axiomatic that handicapped children should be sent to ordinary schools 'whenever possible'. It would be better to say: 'whenever it is in the child's best interest'. If a child in an ordinary school with the 'best available' help is failing educationally, socially and emotionally, it would be in his best interest that he should move (perhaps only temporarily) to a special school for children with epilepsy where he would be a first class citizen, rather than that he should stay on as a third class citizen to satisfy some latter day shibboleth.

General advice

Children with epilepsy are not monsters with forked tails. They are just children, and advice about bringing them up is much the same as advice about bringing up any child. However, the epileptic child does have potential problems and certain commonsensical advice needs to be emphasized.

1. Attitude to epilepsy

Children at school are much more likely to be cruel to each other than are adults at work (Ch.9). However, children are particularly likely to reflect the attitudes of others. If the teacher understands epilepsy and accepts fits in a matter of fact way, and if the child has learnt to adjust to and cope with his epilepsy, the other children will consider him no more unusual than that other child with the leg iron. If he is persecuted it will be because they find him a nasty little boy and not because he has fits.

A child needs to be educated about his fits in much the same way as an older child is about the facts of life. His fits will surprise and mystify him. He will ask questions which should be answered simply and openly. If he has complex partial seizures without full loss of consciousness, he may be frightened and yet unable to express his fear. He will need reassurance. Understanding and adjustment will develop gradually as the child grows up, and he will learn to deal in a natural way with an unnatural event. It would be to lose credibility to dismiss seizures as nothing to worry about. A young child may pay no more attention to his psychic clothes (p. 119) than to those others left strewn around the floor, but when his fragile self image is shattered by the consequences of a seizure, it will take all his mother's skill to re-dress him.

2. Attitude to others

Children who have had fits from an early age and who have some brain damage will have difficulty not only in formal school learning but in learning social skills—not social etiquette but how to get on with other people. They are not incapable of learning, but they take longer, and parents must have the patience and understanding to help them. It can help to play through situations of potential difficulty and even offer the vulnerable child a handbook of useful comments. For example, to the over protective teacher fussing after he has had a fit: 'Thank you very much, really I can manage, I always do, and now I would like to get on with my lessons.' To that other child who is starting to persecute: 'I feel sorry for you. You say silly things because you do not understand.'

3. The doctor

Well before the child is due to go to school the parents should have a full discussion with the responsible doctor—family doctor or paediatrician—and get from him detailed instructions to be passed on to the school. It is helpful if they can be written down: what restrictions, if any, do his particular type of fit require; how should the fit itself be managed; how long should he be allowed to recover; should any side effects be expected from the drugs he is taking; under what circumstances should the doctor be called? The parents probably know the answers to all these questions but the school is much more likely to accept medical instruction than parental interference. Although children metabolize antiepileptic drugs more quickly it is often possible to give the drug in morning and evening doses and so avoid the embarrassment of having to take pills at school. If the doctor has not already arranged this, the parents can ask about it.

4. The headmistress (or headmaster)

The parents should now visit the head of the school, provided, if possible, with the doctor's written instructions. They can fill in further details and emphasize particular points: the importance of keeping restrictions to the minimum, little premonitory signs which may warn the teacher that a fit is coming, the maximum time that the child needs to recover, the use of special equipment if there is incontinence and arrangements for disposing of it.

As long as the parents are talking about their own child they are in a position to tell the teacher, particularly if they have their doctor's support. If they are dealing with a headmistress who has had experience of epilepsy and the correct attitude to its management, they must avoid irritating her by giving a general dissertation. If they are up against old fashioned ideas it may be possible for them to suggest that the children in the school might benefit from a talk on epilepsy given by an experienced speaker from one of the Epilepsy Associations.

Although tonic-clonic seizures may be alarming, it is easy for the school to adapt to them provided that they do not feel anxious and insecure from lack of instruction on what action is needed. Simple or complex absences and other complex partial seizures often create much greater problems and need to be explained fully to both teachers and the other children.

Even if the child only has seizures at night it is necessary to discuss his epilepsy with the school. It is possible that the pattern of attacks might change, and a child's school performance is often impaired the morning after a severe nocturnal seizure.

Later, when the child has started school, the parents should keep in close touch. Difficulties at school or at home can be discussed; the school can report on the number of fits and the parents on any change in treatment or observations from the doctor. If the parents have been sensible enough to follow this advice so far, they will be sensible enough to realise that, while they have one child with epilepsy and problems, the school has 99 children without epilepsy and with problems.

5. Independence

Parents need to protect their children but in parallel they are training them to increase their independence: doing up buttons, zipping up zips and tying up shoe-laces. The child with epilepsy will need, of course, to be taught these things, but also how to deal with his fits, with incontinence, how to explain about epilepsy to other children, and how to deal with good natured teasing without over-reacting and thinking he is being picked on because he has fits. Because the child may be slow to learn, that is will take more time to learn, this does not mean that he cannot learn. It is all too easy for parents to be over-protective and prolong his dependence because they feel he is incapable of independence. Any counsellor must make sure that the parents are encouraging the appropriate degree of independence. Does he use public transport? Perhaps the mother really cannot face such a move. It would help if the child carried an Epilepsy Association card in his pocket or wore a Medicalert bracelet. Perhaps, at first a friend would not mind travelling unobtrusively the same route as the child. The child should be taught how to use a public telephone and given a special reserve of money to use it. From an early stage he can learn that it is good manners and considerate to let his family know if for any reason he has been delayed.

6. Achievement and approval

One of the most important stimuli to effort is the personal sense of achievement and the public approval of a job well done. The child with epilepsy who may have a slight degree of mental handicap needs not only sympathy, understanding and support, but perhaps more importantly the opportunity to achieve genuine success at something within his capability, to merit not patronage but genuine praise. This applies particularly to a child from an intelligent and sophisticated family.

Certainly he will be surrounded by well-structured enlightenment, but it is much more difficult for him to feel that he plays a positive role in the life of the family. The same principle applies at school. If a child is so handicapped that despite his best efforts he never has the chance of success or experiences the joy of spontaneous praise, might he not be better in another school with children of equal handicap? There is no simple answer.

14

Second childhood

Certain aspects of fits and epilepsy which are particular to old people are worth summarizing. In some ways the reactions of the failing body and brain of ancients may be compared with those of the immature body and brain of infants. The brain sensitivity is low but there are more occasions of brain damage. Control of the internal environment is less efficient and its abnormalities may lead to fits, if not to epilepsy. Drugs are metabolized more slowly. Fits are often atypical and there are other conditions with which they may be confused.

Brain sensitivity

Old age is a time when brain sensitivity seems to be damped down.

1. People who have had seizures all their lives often find that as they get older their seizures become less frequent and that they may stop altogether in old age. Even if partial attacks continue, they are less likely to become generalized.

2. If fits start in old age they are much more likely to be partial seizures.

Brain damage

Brain damage is common in old age. Often it is patchy and imperceptibly progressive due to:

1. Vascular (blood vessel) disease (p. 16).
2. Atrophy or loss of brain substance (p. 17).

Failure to control the internal environment

Important changes in the body fluids which surround the nerve cells of the brain, if associated with a degree of brain sensitivity or of brain damage, will precipitate fits. The ageing body is less capable of controlling its own internal environment. For example:

1. disturbances of heart rate (p. 7)
2. failure of the kidney to get rid of harmful waste products (p. 8).

Drug metabolism

Doctors should review the antiepileptic drugs of their older patients with a view to making appropriate reductions.

1. Old people (like the very young) metabolize drugs more slowly.
2. The aged brain, particularly if the site of many small zones of brain damage, is sensitive to drugs, and ill effects appear at serum levels considered suitable for a younger person.
3. Brain sensitivity and the liability to fits are reduced as people get older.

Old people are subject to all sorts of general illnesses which impair further the body's metabolic capability. When they fall ill any possible evidence of intoxication, such as confusion or drowsiness, should be reported to the doctor.

Diagnostic difficulties

Some of the conditions which can be confused with epilepsy are dealt with in Chapter 3 (p. 51). Many of these affect the old. However, there are many occasions when one cannot be sure. There is an event. Doctors should not worry too much. Is it a fit? Is it epilepsy? Is it brain dysfunction due to lack of blood? How much is brain sensitivity? How much is brain damage? How much is loss of control of the internal environment? They do better when their concern is more for their patient's general welfare than for semantics. Three principles should be followed when dealing with fits (or not) at the end of life.

1. Seek out and treat as far as possible any general condition which may be affecting the patient's internal environment.

2. Give the least possible dose of antiepileptic drugs. Partial seizures tend to be very resistant to drugs and, if the patient is showing no signs of the development of generalized attacks, some doctors would withhold antiepileptic drugs altogether.

3. Do not carry out investigations unless there is some prospect of finding a condition which can be treated. For example, the EEG is very seldom useful in the case of elderly patients who have had partial attacks. Nevertheless, a great many are subjected to lying still for half an hour on a hard couch with an even harder pillow under their head, surrounded by apparatus terrifying to those not conditioned to space age television.

Throughout this book our theme has been that epilepsy is not a diagnosis of doom and disaster: sometimes just a nuisance, sometimes a distinct disadvantage, occasionally a disability: that people with epilepsy are people just like other people. Towards the end of their lives, the management of their seizures becomes less of a problem and they become overtaken by the problems of getting old. Like all old people they can be helped best by sympathy and wise understanding.

Glossary

Abscess
A collection of infected matter as in a large boil. Brain abscesses are particularly likely to cause seizures.

Air encephalogram
A technique for visualising the spaces in the brain occupied by csf. A lumbar puncture is carried out, csf is withdrawn and replaced by air. X-rays are taken.

Alpha rhythm
Normal waves recorded on the EEG from the back of the head. Voltage changes of around 50 microvolts occur roughly 10 times a second. The changes get less when the patient is alerted, as when he opens his eyes.

Amnesia
Loss of memory.

Artefacts
In EEG work electrical changes which are recorded as a result of events other than those in the brain. They are confusing and may be difficult to differentiate from true brain waves.

Arteriogram
A technique for visualizing the blood vessels of the brain. X-rays are taken at intervals after the injection of a radio-opaque dye.

Atrophy
Loss of substance. In the very old the brain tends to shrivel up or atrophy.

Aura
A warning that a seizure is coming on. In fact the aura is the very beginning of a partial seizure of which the patient is aware because he has not lost consciousness. Some patients have frequent aurae which do not develop any further.

Autonomic nervous system
Those nerves which control the working of the internal organs and maintain a suitable internal environment. It is not under direct voluntary control nor do most of its activities impinge on consciousness.

Axons
Fibres which carry messages to or from the nerve cell.

Cerebral
To do with that part of the brain which is developed enormously in man in the form of two hemispheres which lie at the top of the brain stem.

Cerebrospinal fluid (CSF)
Fluid lying in spaces within and on the surface of the brain. A specimen can be withdrawn for examination by lumbar puncture.

Channel
In EEG work each line on the record is referred to as a channel. A channel records the electrical changes between the two electrodes to which it is connected.

Clonic phase
That part of a seizure during which there is jerking resulting from alternate contraction and relaxation of muscles.

Coma
Deep unconsciousness when the patient makes little or no response to stimuli.

Complex absence
A slight complex partial seizure in which there is loss or alteration of consciousness with few other features. It usually lasts longer than a simple absence and is associated with some other features of a complex partial seizure. The two can be distinguished by the EEG.

Compliance
A term used to describe the extent to which a patient takes the drugs prescribed by his doctor.

Computerized tomography (CT scan)
A technique in which large numbers of x-rays of the brain provide brain maps at different planes.

Cortex
The layer of nerve cells on the surface of the brain, seen as up to four millimetres of grey matter.

Cyanosis
A dark bluish colour of the skin, lips and nail beds due to lack of oxygen in the blood. There may be severe cyanosis when breathing stops during the tonic phase of a tonic-clonic convulsion.

Déjà vu
A feeling that what is happening has all happened before. Normal people sometimes have such feelings. When they are overwhelming, they suggest the aura of a complex partial seizure.

Dementia
Impairment of intellectual function. Commonly this arises insiduously and progressively in older people and is due to loss of brain substance from disease or atrophy.

Dendrites
Processes of the nerve cell which receive messages from other nerve cells.

Differential diagnosis
Possible causes of a condition, e.g. the differential diagnosis of sudden loss of consciousness would include: a faint, an epileptic seizure and severe disturbance of the heart beat.

ECT (electroconvulsive therapy)
Seizures are provoked by passing electric currents through the brain. Useful in mental illness, particularly depression.

EEG (electroencephalograph)
A recording of the electrical changes in the brain which have been amplified several million times.

Electrode
In EEG work the pads or discs placed on the scalp to make electrical contact.

Embolism
The blockage of a blood vessel by a clot, which has formed elsewhere, and has been carried in the blood stream.

Encephalitis
An infection of the brain substance.

Febrile convulsions
Seizures, usually tonic-clonic convulsions, occurring in small children when they have a high temperature due to an infection.

Grey matter
Those parts of the brain and the spinal cord where there are collections of nerve cells. They appear darker than white matter because the nerve cells have a more plentiful blood supply.

Gyrus (pl. gyri)
Ridges seen on the surface of the brain.

Haematoma
A collection of blood as a result of a bleed.

Haemorrhage
A bleed.

Hallucination
An imagined sensory experience for which there is no real basis. e.g. Hearing voices, which are not there, talking to you.

Hypoglycaemia
Too little sugar in the blood, as for example after too much insulin.

Hysteria (hysterical reaction)
In psychological terms, a condition in which a patient, faced with a situation with which he cannot cope, unconsciously develops symptoms of disease. Hysterical fits may occur in patients who also have epileptic fits.

Idiopathic epilepsy
Epilepsy for which no cause can be found. It does not mean that there is no brain damage, only that none can be found. A term not used much nowadays.

Incontinent

Not able to control or contain. During a seizure it is common for a patient to pass water involuntarily—to be incontinent of urine. Faecal incontinence is less common.

Jamais vu

A distortion of perception, which may occur as the aura of a complex partial seizure, in which familiar objects appear strange.

Lesion

Damage caused by disease or injury.

Lobe

Zones into which the cerebral hemispheres are divided.

Lumbar puncture

A technique for obtaining a specimen of csf by inserting a long needle between the bones of the lower spine into the space surrounding the nerves leading from the bottom of the spinal cord.

Medilog

A system in which the EEG can be recorded on cassettes continuously over long periods while the patient carries on his normal activities.

Meninges

The membranes which cover the brain. The dura is the thick protective outer covering. The arachnoid is thinner and whispy like a spider's web where small blood vessel ramify before they supply the brain. See also: subdural haematoma and subarachnoid haemorrhage.

Meningitis

An infection of the meninges.

Metabolism

Chemical changes usually carried out by the liver. The body treats antepileptic drugs as foreign substances and metabolises them so that they can be got rid of more easily.

Microvolt

One millionth part of a volt. The electrical changes in the brain are so small that they are measured in microvolts.

Micturate (micturition)

Pass water.

Motor nerves

Nerves which carry instructions to muscles.

Myoclonus (myoclonic)

A sudden muscle contraction producing a jerk. It may be due to severe brain damage, or be a manifestation of primary generalized seizures. Normal people often have occasional myoclonic jerks as they are falling asleep.

Occipital

The lobes at the back of the brain. They are concerned in part with the reception of vision.

Paranoia
A severe form of mental illness (psychosis) in which the patient holds a fixed and incorrect belief which cannot be shaken by the most convincing evidence that it is incorrect, e.g. he may feel that everyone is against him and is plotting to poison him.

Paroxysmal abnormality
In EEG work a sudden change in the record. If a patient has attacks of loss of consciousness, and if his EEG shows paroxysms, it is likely that the attacks are epileptic. If an observed change in behaviour, is accompanied by a paroxysmal EEG abnormality, it is highly probable that the patient has had some form of seizure.

Photophobia
Intolerance of light. Found when the surface of the brain is irritated whether by an infection (meningitis) or a bleed (subarachnoid haemorrhage).

Post-central
Concerning the gyrus which lies behind the main central sulcus. It receives sensory information from the opposite side of the body.

Post-traumatic
After injury. e.g. post-traumatic amnesia, loss of memory for a period after a head injury.

Pre-central
Concerning the gyrus which lies in front of the main central sulcus. It initiates simple movements of the opposite side of the body.

Prodromal
Relating to rather vague symptoms which may appear for hours or even days before a seizure. Prodromal symptoms should be distinguished from the aura which is the early part of a partial seizure before consciousness is affected.

Prognosis
An estimate of what is going to happen. If a patient is given a good prognosis, he is likely to get better.

Psychosis
A severe form of mental illness.

Sensory nerves
Nerves which carry information to the spinal cord, or, in the case of special senses such as sight, to the brain.

Serial seizures
When there are frequent seizures, one after another, but with recovery of consciousness in between.

Serum level
The amount of substance in the blood.

Sharp wave
In EEG work, a change in the electricity in the brain, less rapid than that producing a spike, causes a rather less pointed deflection.

Simple absence (petit mal)
A very mild form of primary generalized seizure, nearly always affecting children, which is less common that it was thought to be.

Spikes
In EEG work, when there is a very rapid change in electricity in the brain, the very pointed deflection is referred to as a spike.

Status epilepticus
When one seizure follows another without recovery of consciousness in between. Usually referred to just as 'status'.

Subarachnoid haemorrhage
Bleeding under the arachnoid, a thin whispy membrane covering the brain. Usually due to the bursting of a blood vessel. Sudden and quite often fatal.

Sulcus (pl. sulci)
Folds in the cortex of the cerebral hemispheres. This infolding increases a great deal the surface area of the cortex.

Symptomatic epilepsy
Epilepsy caused by some proven brain damage. A term not used much nowadays.

Syncope
Loss of consciousness due to failure of the blood supply to the brain.

Temporal
The lobe at the side of the brain which lies beneath the temple. Damage to part of the temporal lobe results in complex partial seizures (sometimes called temporal lobe epilepsy), one of the commonest types of epilepsy.

Thrombosis
Blockage of a blood vessel.

Tonic-clonic convulsion (grand mal)
A severe seizure which may be primary or may develop from a simple or complex partial seizure.

Tonic phase
That phase of a tonic-clonic convulsion when muscles are held in steady contraction. Breathing will stop and, if the tonic phase is long, there will be deep cyanosis.

Tumour
A lump or growth. A term associated in people's minds with cancer. In fact most tumours are harmless or benign.

Vascular
To do with blood vessels.

White matter
Those parts of the brain and spinal cord where nerve fibres are grouped together. They look white because the fibres are covered with a white fatty substance.

Appendix A

Official or generic name	Best known proprietary name	Tablet size	
carbamazepine	Tegretol	100/200/400 mg	Main drugs in
phenytoin	Epanutin	50/100 mg	general use.
		25/50/100 mg	
		(caps)	
sodium valproate	Epilim	200/500 mg	
ethosuximide	Zarontin	250 mg	Drugs now used
phenobarbitone	Luminal	15/30/60/100 mg	less often.
primidone	Mysoline	250 mg	
acetazolamide	Diamox	250 mg	Drugs now
		500 mg (caps)	seldom used.
beclamide	Nydrane	500 mg	
sulthiame	Ospolot	50/200	
troxidone	Tridione	300 mg	
clobazam	Frisium	10 mg	Drug recently introduced for epilepsy.
clonazepam	Rivotril	0.5 mg & 2 mg	Drugs used for
diazepam	Valium	2/5/10 mg	special
nitrazepam	Mogadon	5 mg	purposes.

Phenytoin is marketed as Dilantin in Australia, Canada, New Zealand and the U.S.A.

Sodium valproate is marketed as Depakene in the U.S.A. and by a variety of other names in Europe.

Most of these drugs are available in liquid form for young children and those unable to take tablets.

Appendix B

NAMES AND ADDRESSES OF THE EPILEPSY ASSOCIATIONS IN THE UNITED KINGDOM

These Associations provide a very useful information service and should be consulted for up to date legislation about Driving Licences and also such practical matters as immigration restrictions and the names and addresses of foreign Epilepsy Associations.

British Epilepsy Association,
Room 16,
Claremont Street Hospital,
Belfast BT9 6AQ.
(0232) 40491 ext. 23

British Epilepsy Association,
1st Floor—Guildhall Buildings,
Navigation Street,
Birmingham, B2 4BT.
(021) 643 7524

Mersey Region Epilepsy Association,
138 The Albany,
Old Hall Street,
Liverpool, L3 9EY.
(051) 263 0990

British Epilepsy Association,
North Regional Centre,
313 Chapeltown Road,
Leeds, LS7 3JT.
(0532) 621076

British Epilepsy Association,
Crowthorne House
New Wokingham Road,
Wokingham, Berkshire, RG11 3AY.
(034 46) 3122

The Epilepsy Association of Scotland:

CENTRAL
255 Main Street,
Larbert, FK5.
0324-553347.

STRATHCLYDE
48 Govan Road,
Glasgow, G51 1JL.
041-427-4911

GRAMPIAN
14 Turnberry Cr.,
Bridge of Don,
Aberdeen.
0224-868801.

TAYSIDE
35 Woodmuir Terrace,
Newport on Tay.
0382-542383.

LOTHIAN
13 Guthrie Street,
Edinburgh, EH1 1JG.
031-226-5458.

The National Society for Epilepsy,
Chalfont Centre for Epilepsy,
Chalfont St, Peter,
Gerrards Cross,
Buckinghamshire. SL9 0RJ.
(024 07) 3991
Provides a valuable information service.

MEDICALERT BRACELET OR NECKLET

The Medicalert Foundation, 9 Hanover Street, London W1R 9HF
For a small fee this foundation provides a useful service to those liable to a medical emergency, in this case epilepsy. The patient wears either a bracelet or a necklet on which is inscribed his medical problem (epilepsy) his personal serial number and an emergency telephone number. This number may be called (the charges being reversed) by any authorised person and information provided by the patient's own doctor is given from the central file.

Index

Page numbers in bold indicate principal references; (g) indicates that the entry appears in the glossary.